Ella Simpson
January 2020

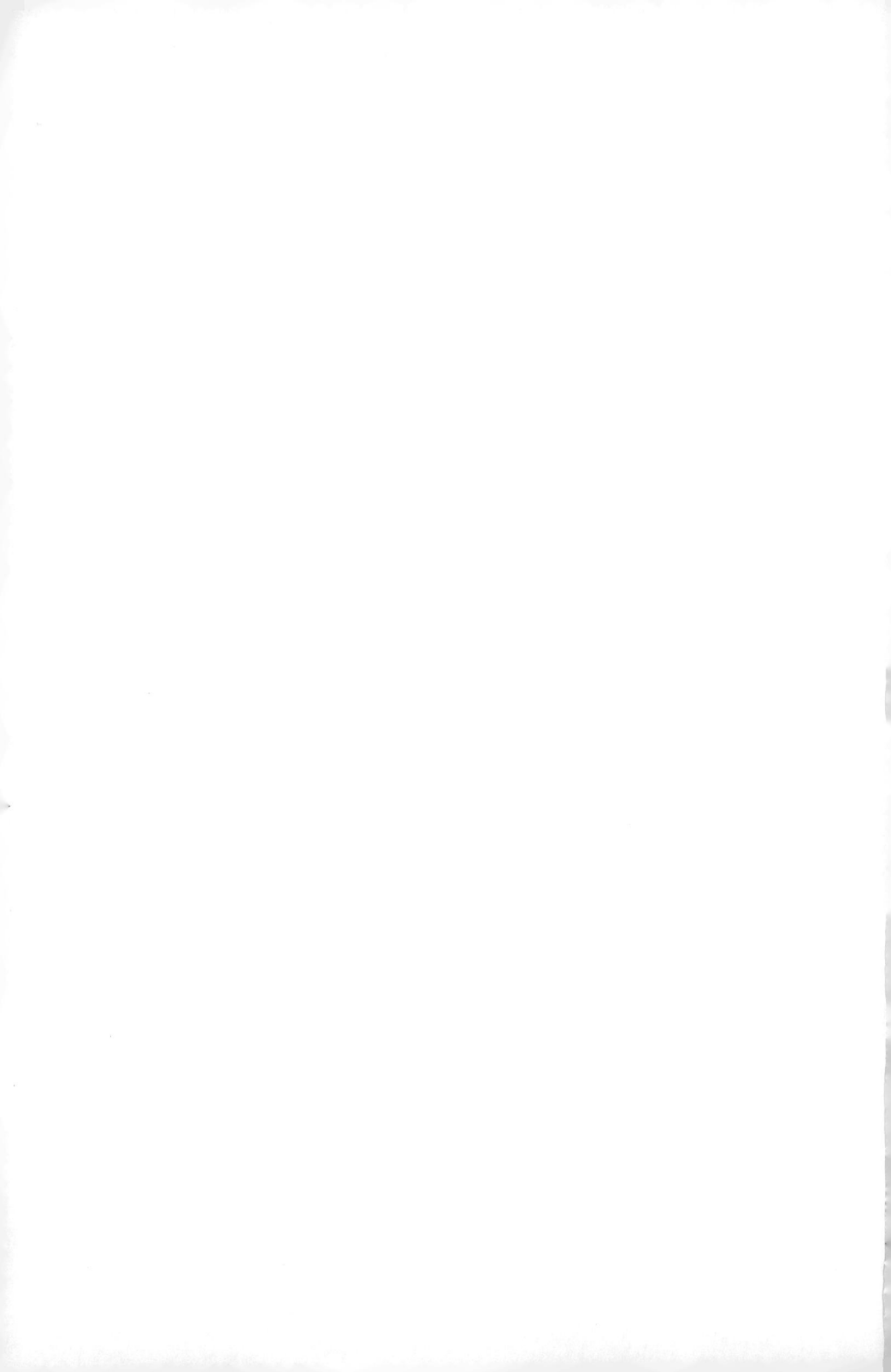

Midwifery, Childbirth and the Media

Ann Luce · Vanora Hundley
Edwin van Teijlingen
Editors

Midwifery, Childbirth and the Media

palgrave
macmillan

Editors
Ann Luce
Bournemouth University
Bournemouth, UK

Vanora Hundley
Bournemouth University
Bournemouth, UK

Edwin van Teijlingen
Centre for Midwifery, Maternal
 and Perinatal Health
Bournemouth University
Bournemouth, UK

ISBN 978-3-319-63512-5   ISBN 978-3-319-63513-2   (eBook)
DOI 10.1007/978-3-319-63513-2

Library of Congress Control Number: 2017950679

© The Editor(s) (if applicable) and The Author(s) 2017
This work is subject to copyright. All rights are solely and exclusively licensed by the Publisher, whether the whole or part of the material is concerned, specifically the rights of translation, reprinting, reuse of illustrations, recitation, broadcasting, reproduction on microfilms or in any other physical way, and transmission or information storage and retrieval, electronic adaptation, computer software, or by similar or dissimilar methodology now known or hereafter developed.
The use of general descriptive names, registered names, trademarks, service marks, etc. in this publication does not imply, even in the absence of a specific statement, that such names are exempt from the relevant protective laws and regulations and therefore free for general use.
The publisher, the authors and the editors are safe to assume that the advice and information in this book are believed to be true and accurate at the date of publication. Neither the publisher nor the authors or the editors give a warranty, express or implied, with respect to the material contained herein or for any errors or omissions that may have been made. The publisher remains neutral with regard to jurisdictional claims in published maps and institutional affiliations.

Cover illustration: © Melisa Hasan

Printed on acid-free paper

This Palgrave Macmillan imprint is published by Springer Nature
The registered company is Springer International Publishing AG
The registered company address is: Gewerbestrasse 11, 6330 Cham, Switzerland

Contents

1. Introduction   1
   Ann Luce, Vanora Hundley and Edwin van Teijlingen

2. Love Birth, Hate *One Born Every Minute?* Birth Community Discourse Around Televised Childbirth   7
   Julie Roberts, Sara De Benedictis and Helen Spiby

3. Birth Stories in British Newspapers: Why Midwives Must Speak up   23
   Emily Maclean

4. An Everyday Trauma: How the Media Portrays Infant Feeding   45
   Catherine Angell

5. How Media Promote Fear Around Childbirth   61
   Alexia Leachman

6. 'Passing Time': A Qualitative Study of Health Promotion Practices in an Antenatal Clinic Waiting Room   79
   Dianne Rodger, Andrew Skuse and Michael Wilmore

7	**Midwives' Engagement with the Media** Ann Luce, Vanora Hundley, Edwin van Teijlingen, Sian Ridden and Sofie Edlund	97
8	**Working With the Media: The Power, the Pitfalls and the Possibilities** Hannah G. Dahlen	111
9	**Around the World in 80 Tweets—Social Media and Midwifery** Sheena Byrom and Anna Byrom	129
Conclusions		149
Index		153

EDITORS AND CONTRIBUTORS

About the Editors

Dr. Ann Luce is a Principal Academic in Journalism and Communication at Bournemouth University. A journalist-turned-academic, she is working with midwives on changing the discourses around midwifery in the media. Other research she has conducted focuses on teaching disabled people how to become citizen journalists and she is the recent author of, "The Bridgend Suicides: Suicide and the Media".

Prof. Vanora Hundley is Professor of Midwifery in the Centre for Midwifery, Maternal and Perinatal Health at Bournemouth University. She has published widely in the field of midwifery and maternal health. She is Associate Editor for BMC Pregnancy and Childbirth.

Prof. Edwin van Teijlingen is a medical sociologist based in the Centre for Midwifery, Maternal and Perinatal Health at Bournemouth University. He is co-editor of books on health/maternity care published with Routledge, Oxford University Press and NOVA (New York). He is Associate Editor for BMC Pregnancy and Childbirth.

Contributors

Dr. Catherine Angell is a Principal Academic in Midwifery in the Centre for Midwifery, Maternal and Perinatal Health at Bournemouth University. Her research interests include education, breastfeeding and media representation of maternity care.

Sheena Byrom OBE was one of the United Kingdom's first consultant midwives. She is a board member of the Royal College of Midwives and Chair of the Iolanthe Midwifery Trust. She is a well-known blogger in the midwifery field and can be found on Twitter @sagefemmeSB.

Anna Byrom is a Lecturer and Ph.D. Student at the University of Central Lancashire in the School of Community Health and Midwifery. She is a member of Progress Theatre, a midwifery theatre company who deliver interactive workshops around the United Kingdom relating to specific issues in maternity care provision.

Hannah G. Dahlen is Professor of Midwifery at Western Sydney University. She has been a midwife for more than 25 years. She is also an executive member of the Australian College of Midwives, NSW Branch. She has researched women's birth experiences at home and in hospital and published extensively in this area.

She is a leading midwifery researcher in Australia, with an international reputation as an outstanding midwifery scholar. This is demonstrated through publication of over 120 papers and book chapters, presentation of over 100 conference papers, more than half being invited keynote addresses (16 international keynotes, 50 national) and strong international collaborations. Hannah has been interviewed on TV, radio and in newspapers and magazines over 1,000 times in her career. She has been involved in three documentaries about childbirth (*Face of Birth*, *Microbirth* and *Hannah's Story*) In November 2012 she was named in the *Sydney Morning Herald*'s list of 100 "people who change our city for the better" as one of the leading "science and knowledge thinkers" due to her research and public profile. She is one of the leading writers for *The Conversation*, where research is explained in a way that is accessible to lay people.

Dr. Sara De Benedictis explores the representation of birth in British reality television programmes. She has worked for a number of UK women's organisations in the third sector. She completed a post-doc at The University of Nottingham.

Sofie Edlund was a final-year undergraduate student at Bournemouth University studying for a degree in Communication and Media. She conducted her research with the help of the Centre for Excellence in Learning at Bournemouth University.

Alexia Leachman is the host of the 'Fear Free Childbirth' podcast that is listened to in over 100 countries and has been downloaded more than 70,000 times in the last year. She is also a digital brand strategist and a coach. She is due to release her second book, *Fearless Birthing*, in 2016.

Emily Maclean is a former journalist who trained at the *Daily Mirror* before working as a freelance correspondent across Africa for a range of British national newspapers. Now a midwife, she is engaged in media campaigns with the Royal College of Midwives, writes in academic and news publications, and is a peer reviewer for Midwifery and the British Journal of Midwifery. Her background includes an M.Sc in Public Health at the London School of Hygiene and Tropical Medicine, an M.A. in Modern Languages at the University of Oxford and a course in Qualitative Research Methods, also at Oxford.

Sian Ridden was a midwifery student at Bournemouth University and is now a practicing midwife. She conducted her research with the help of the Centre for Excellence in Learning at Bournemouth University.

Dr. Julie Roberts is a sociologist and qualitative researcher interested in the social context of pregnancy and birth. She has published widely on cultural representations of ultrasound images and experiences of health.

Dr. Dianne Rodger is an anthropologist whose research interests include popular culture, music and communication. She is an early-career researcher with growing specialisation in the areas of youth culture, sub-cultural research and media consumption (in particular the use of new technologies such as social media). She was the Senior Research Fellow on the Health-e Baby project and is currently employed as a Lecturer at the University of Adelaide.

Prof. Andrew Skuse is Head of the Department of Anthropology and Development Studies and manages the Applied Communication Collaborative Research Unit (ACCRU) at the University of Adelaide,

South Australia. His research and professional work focuses on how poor and vulnerable people interact with information and communication technologies and how these may positively affect livelihoods, health, education, peace-building and social equity.

Prof. Helen Spiby is a midwife with longstanding research interests in preparation for and care during labour. Recent studies mapped how antenatal preparation is provided through NHS maternity services and explored families' expectations and experiences of preparation for labour.

Prof. Michael Wilmore's research encompasses the disciplines of media and anthropology. He has worked on projects in Nepal, Australia and the United Kingdom, investigating issues in development and health communication. He has also held a number of faculty leadership roles supporting learning and teaching, and is currently Executive Dean of the Faculty of Media and Communication, Bournemouth University.

List of Tables

Table 8.1	Five key elements constitute a series of core oppositions	117
Table 9.1	Social media platforms and application examples	132
Table 9.2	Frequency of use on social media sites (Pew 2015)	133
Table 9.3	Glossary of social media terms	135
Table 9.4	Benefits of social media for knowledge translation	139
Table 9.5	Key social media platforms for knowledge translation (KT)	140

CHAPTER 1

Introduction

Ann Luce, Vanora Hundley and Edwin van Teijlingen

Abstract The media plays an important role in providing us with information about a range of topics and issues, including pregnancy and childbirth. The visual media, such as television, can provide planned information (education), for example, in documentaries, advertising and the news. But the information can also be unplanned (through socialisation), for example, through the way issues are portrayed in soap operas, "fly-on-the-wall" programs, panel shows and drama. There has been a considerable debate regarding the influence the media has on first-time pregnant women. Much of the academic literature discusses the influence of (reality) television, which often portrays childbirth as risky, dramatic and painful. The truth is that most of pregnancy and childbirth is slow, relatively 'uneventful', and marked by long periods of waiting. Therefore, normal childbirth is not great for visual media such as television. There is anecdotal evidence to suggest that the dramatic portrayal

---

A. Luce (✉) · V. Hundley · E. van Teijlingen
Bournemouth University, Bournemouth, UK
e-mail: aluce@bournemouth.ac.uk

V. Hundley
e-mail: vhundley@bournemouth.ac.uk

E. van Teijlingen
e-mail: evteijlingen@bournemouth.ac.uk

of childbirth has a negative effect on childbirth in society, generating fear of childbirth through the increasing anticipation of negative outcomes. At the same time, it has been suggested that women seek out such programmes to help understand what could happen during the birth. This chapter will introduce the current thinking by health professionals about the role of media in how women perceive birth.

Keywords Media · Midwifery · Debate · Childbirth · Early labour

When we came together as a research team back in 2013, little had been written about the media's role in early labour and childbirth. We knew that many high-income countries were experiencing rising rates of childbirth interventions with little evidence that those interventions lead to improvements in maternal or newborn outcomes (EURO-PERISTAT 2013). We knew that explanatory factors for the rise in interventions included negative birth experiences, cultural perceptions and societal attitudes that influenced women's decisions about when to enter hospital in labour; and we hypothesised that the way in which childbirth is portrayed by the media could lead to fear and anxiety about the birthing process, thus also having an impact. Fear is increasingly cited as a reason for rising rates of intervention in childbirth and the reason that some women opt for a caesarean section rather than going through a natural labour (Hundley et al. 2014).

To test these assumptions, we held a debate at Bournemouth University in 2014. The debate sparked a heated discussion amongst midwives in attendance, but a point raised by our media colleagues made us stop and think. They argued that the responsibility for balanced reporting of childbirth lay not with the media, but with the midwifery profession. Midwives, they said, needed to harness the power of the media to change discourse; midwives needed to be more media-savvy.

Midwives frequently state that media portrayals of childbirth are dramatic, focus on the risks and are just simply unrealistic; normal birth is not shown. We conducted a scoping review to identify how childbirth is represented in the mass media, and in particular, television (Luce et al. 2016). In that review, we found 56 publications met our inclusion criteria: (a) published in English, (b) included research (qualitative, quantitative or mixed-methods approach) and (c) contained portrayals of childbirth and/or labour in the media. After duplicates, opinion pieces and student essays were eliminated, we were left with 12 qualitative and 5 quantitative studies; 3 unpublished research pieces and 18 elements of grey literature, which included papers from professional journals, conference proceedings, on-line discussion forums and a book chapter. Key themes that emerged from the literature were (a) the medicalization of childbirth, (b) women using media to learn about childbirth and (c) birth as a missing everyday life event. According to Hundley et al. (2015), "it was clear from the literature that birth is frequently portrayed by the media as fast, furious and carrying such significant medical risk that women must rush immediately to hospital when labour begins" (7). What was noticeable by its absence was any evidence about the effect that such representations have on women and the health professionals that care for them.

Midwives blame the media for these misrepresentations of childbirth, yet we have argued elsewhere that we believe that midwives have a responsibility to engage with media producers and journalists when it comes to childbirth and early labour. Little research has been conducted that engages with media producers to try and understand their production processes and why they present stories and storylines in the way that they do. We believe that midwives can harness the media to get positive messages into the public sphere; however, to do this it is important that we have an understanding of how the media works and the impact it can have on pregnant women and the midwifery profession. Midwives have a critical role to play within the media, and this includes harnessing the power of social media.

The challenge we face is that we are dealing with two independent professions who both think they have ownership over how midwifery and childbirth should be represented in the media. In order to change the narrative around birth these two fields must be brought together; there must be discussion and collaboration. With this in mind, we have brought together a group of leading international scholars in both fields to help explain the complexities of the research that has been completed and identify what still needs to be done. We have loosely broken this book down into three sections: portrayals in the media and the effects of those portrayals, the midwife response and how to engage with media.

In the first section on *Portrayals in the Media and the Effects of Those Portrayals*, Julie Roberts, Sara De Benedictis and Helen Spiby at The University of Nottingham discuss the pitfalls around the highly controversial *One Born Every Minute (Channel 4, 2010)* in Chap. 2.

They question if OBEM should be banned? Is it educational? Does it instil fear in pregnant women? The authors take us through an in-depth reading of this show, asking whether it is possible to achieve the "perfect representation of birth." In Chap. 3, Emily Maclean, a journalist turned midwife explores the representation of midwifery in British newspapers. Using her own experience as a journalist to help underpin her arguments, Maclean discusses the types of birth stories reported in newspapers and how headlines continue to portray birth as an extreme event, yet she claims there is space for "normal" birth stories, too. She explores this and offers suggestions for how midwives can help in providing access and change the story narrative. In Chap. 4, Catherine Angell, a senior academic in midwifery at Bournemouth University, takes us through an in-depth study looking at representations of infant feeding in British newspapers from 1999 to 2016. She discusses media messages, stereotyping and whether breastfeeding is considered an "ordinary or extraordinary" event. She highlights the confusion that occurs when the media provides entertainment through drama and tragedy and the impact that has on a woman's birth experience and motherhood. Alexia Leachman, creator of the *Fear Free Childbirth Podcast* rounds, out this section in Chap. 5 with a first-hand narrative account of her own difficulties with childbirth, and how that led to her supporting thousands of women the world over to create positive childbirth environments for themselves and their babies. She provides anecdotal evidence, based on her interactions with women, of the role media plays in shaping perceptions about childbirth.

In the second section, *The Midwife's Response*, in Chap. 6 Dianne Rodger, Andrew Skuse and Michael Wilmore discuss how health-promotion strategies are employed in an Antenatal Clinic waiting room in the Northern suburbs of Adelaide, Australia. They suggest how midwives can better engage pregnant women while waiting for appointments, and how this might help support women further during their pregnancy. In Chap. 7, the editors explore midwives' engagement with the media. Based on interviews with a small group of midwives, the authors discuss whether midwives need to engage with media in order to change discourse, if midwives should use social media as part of their role and whether midwives need media training.

In the final section of this book, *How To Engage With Media*, Hannah G. Dahlen, who has been working as the media spokesperson for the Australian College of Midwives for nearly 20 years, provides an in-depth critique and reflection of working with the Australian media. In Chap. 8 she provides a clear outline of how midwives can engage with media across a range of traditional media platforms. In Chap. 9, Sheena and Anna Byrom build upon Dahlen's work and discuss how midwives can and should engage on social media. A beginner's guide for midwives, this chapter encourages midwives to start small and work up to that first 140-character tweet.

In our concluding chapter, we challenge midwives to engage more with media to harness positive messages about the profession of midwifery and also about childbirth and early labour. We also posit where the research in this area needs to go next and provide a roadmap for those scholars who wish to collaborate in this area.

First, however, Julie Roberts, Sara De Benedictis and Helen Spiby will take us through a discussion about birth-community discourse around televised childbirth.

References

EURO-PERISTAT Project. 2013. European Perinatal Health Report: The health and care of pregnant women and their babies in 2010, Inserm, Paris. Web address: http://www.europeristat.com/reports/european-perinatal-health-report-2010.html.
Hundley, V., E. Duff, J. Dewberry, A. Luce, and E. van Teijlingen. 2014. Fear in childbirth: Are the media responsible? *MIDIRS Midwifery Digest* 24 (4): 444–447.
Hundley, V., E. van Teijlingen, and A. Luce. 2015. Do midwives need to be more media savvy? *MIDIRS Midwifery Digest* 25 (1): 5–10.
Luce, A., M. Cash, M. Hundley, H. Cheyne, E. van Teijlingen, and C. Angell. 2016. "Is it realistic?" The portrayal of pregnancy and childbirth in the media. *BMC Pregnancy and Childbirth*. Accessible Online: https://bmcpregnancychildbirth.biomedcentral.com/articles/10.1186/s12884-016-0827-x.

CHAPTER 2

Love Birth, Hate *One Born Every Minute*? Birth Community Discourse Around Televised Childbirth

Julie Roberts, Sara De Benedictis and Helen Spiby

Abstract Childbirth is highly visible on television at a time when few people see birth in the family or community and access to antenatal education is declining. *One Born Every Minute* (*OBEM*) is the most high-profile example of this programming in the United Kingdom. Now on its ninth series, the series won a BAFTA in its first year and now exports programmes to the United States and France. However, such programming is controversial within the birth community. This chapter examines objections to the series—drawing on an analysis of published commentaries and opinion pieces from midwives, doulas and activists. Firstly we evaluate claims that televised birth promotes fear among women and

J. Roberts (✉) · H. Spiby
University of Nottingham, Nottingham, UK
e-mail: julie.roberts@nottingham.ac.uk

H. Spiby
e-mail: helen.spiby@nottingham.ac.uk

S. De Benedictis
Brunel University London, London, UK
e-mail: Sara.Debenedictis@brunel.ac.uk

© The Author(s) 2017
A. Luce et al. (eds.), *Midwifery, Childbirth and the Media*,
DOI 10.1007/978-3-319-63513-2_2

damages the midwifery profession in the light of available research evidence. Secondly we explore the dominant conceptual questions that emerged from the analysis around the identity of *OBEM* as educational programming or entertainment, and its claims to represent reality. The birth community has raised important questions about birth on television and we draw together insights from a range of disciplines to argue for further research that is theoretically grounded to move the debate forward and tackle the complex question of how televised birth might be influencing women's experiences of pregnancy and birth. The commentaries and opinion pieces from within the 'birth community' raise vital questions about the impact of televised childbirth on women's experiences and on wider birth culture. However, some of the claims identified—that *OBEM* increases fear of birth, that it damages the profession of midwifery—need a stronger empirical basis if they are to be supported. We argue that interdisciplinary, theoretically informed research has potential to further the debate and inform interventions in popular culture.

Keywords *One Born Every Minute* · Television · Childbirth Fear Reality television

Introduction

Childbirth is highly visible on television at a time when few people see birth in the community and access to antenatal education is declining. *One Born Every Minute* (Channel 4, 2010) (*OBEM*) is the most high-profile example of this programming in the United Kingdom. Currently in its ninth series, the series won a BAFTA in its first year and now exports programmes to the United States and France. Until its fourth series, the show regularly attracted 3–4 million viewers (BARB cited in Hamad 2016: 144) and it continues to draw a substantial audience. However, some birth activists and midwives have called for the programme to be banned; others express concern that the programme may have negative social effects on both women and the midwifery profession. As one headline proclaimed: 'Love Birth? You Probably Hate One Born Every Minute' (Hill 2015). This chapter seeks to explore this controversy through a close reading of opinion pieces written by midwives, doulas and birth activists. This somewhat unwieldy group, that we might call the birth community, is made up of those who—in Hill's terms (above)—'love birth'. It connotes a certain expertise in birth and a political engagement with birth in contemporary culture. It is distinguishable from the perspectives of women who have recently given birth, although some of the authors are also mothers. It also does not include obstetricians, from whom we did not identify any similar comment or opinion pieces.

Opinion pieces were found by searching general databases (e.g., LexisNexis), midwifery and obstetrics journals, midwifery activist websites and blogs, birth and doula activist websites and blogs as well as a Google search. These searches identified 33 commentary pieces about *OBEM*. Through close reading of these texts, we identified two common claims made by critics of televised birth: firstly that series like *OBEM* are increasing fear of birth among women, and secondly that the show is harmful to the midwifery profession. We unpick the language and assumptions within these claims and ultimately argue that, although they are valid areas of concern, there is a lack of empirical evidence to support the claims in full. In the second half of the chapter, we move on to two conceptual questions at the heart of the texts: firstly: Is *OBEM* entertainment or education? And secondly: Is it 'real'? We employ our various expertises in the sociology of pregnancy and birth, the analysis of popular representations, and midwifery to explore underlying assumptions that formulate these critiques and how these are shaped through naturalised sociocultural ideas about television, childbirth and knowledge. We contextualise these within the wider field of (reality) television studies. It is in this context that divided views about *OBEM* make sense, as reality television tends to provoke 'fierce reactions' from audiences and commentators and those reactions are often starkly divided (Skeggs and Wood 2012: 2).

Our intention here is not to criticise individuals who draw on their expertise and experience and who passionately advocate for women. Rather, we analyse these opinion pieces as 'discourse'. Discourse comprises 'all forms of talk and texts' that can be analysed to 'draw attention to the fact that discourse is built or manufactured from pre-existing linguistic resources' formed through unequal structural relations; this approach stresses 'discourse as social practice' where 'language is constructive' (Gill 2007: 58, 59). The approach identifies common themes emerging from the texts, highlighting taken-for-granted assumptions. We believe that these underlying assumptions can be analysed with an interdisciplinary lens to produce new insights and tentatively suggest initial steps towards conceptual clarity which we believe may allow the social debate to move forward, both within and outside the birth community, and even inform strategic approaches to intervening in popular culture.

Fear of Childbirth

It is commonly claimed among the birth community that *OBEM*, and shows like it, increase fear of birth among women, particularly first-time mothers:

> The majority I have spoken to are frightened by watching it and yet feel compelled to continue. (Garrod 2012)

> What we may see now is a group of women in their first pregnancy who have a dread of childbirth because of other people's experiences via reality shows. (Barker 2012)

Increased fear is attributed by commentators to the over-representation of highly medicalised births and the reliance of reality television on moments of emergency to add drama to the narrative. In the US context, childbirth educators Lothian and Grauer argue that 'reality shows have made birth appear more medical than ever'; and it is this that is rendering women fearful (Lothian and Grauer 2003: vii).

Tokophobia is considered to be extreme fear of childbirth, although it is poorly defined and rates are hard to determine. Fear of birth is estimated to occur in between 7 and 26% of women in high-income countries (Richens et al. 2015). Fear of childbirth is associated with increased risk of prolonged labour (Laursen et al. 2009; Adams et al. 2012) and emergency Caesarean section (Laursen et al. 2009). Some women avoid planning for birth as a means of coping with fear of childbirth (Fenwick et al. 2015) or choose more medical intervention as a way of managing risk (Greer et al. 2014). As therapist coach and writer Leachman puts it—

> My problem with fear, is that it is directly responsible for crappy childbirth experiences that are bad for mum and bad for baby. (Leachman 2015)

Evidence linking reality television with impacts on women's plans for their childbirth is starting to emerge, although there is relatively little from the UK context.

In many countries, childbirth on television is seen to be fraught with danger. Although the accuracy of depictions has been challenged, it can be difficult to counter when alternatives of straightforward birthing are reported relatively infrequently. There may be other system challenges that reduce women's confidence in their ability to give birth, such as lack of family support during labour or lack of trust in maternity caregivers. In a small study of Canadian women, negative depictions of labour and birth on television have been identified as an influence on requests for caesarean birth in the absence of medical indications (Munro et al. 2009). In a cross-sectional study amongst UK university female students, Thomson and colleagues (2017) identified associations between both what they classified as positive and negative perceptions of birth in visual media with higher ratings of fear of childbirth. However, visual media representations were less influential on fear of childbirth when compared with the negative perceptions of childbirth from family members.

The relationship between media, culture and birth-related behaviour has been underexplored (Luce et al. 2016). Further research is required, including psychosocial and longitudinal approaches, where the impacts of reality television on women's experiences of childbirth can be determined. However, it is no straightforward matter to link televised birth to women's expectations and experiences of birth. Lesley Page, President of the Royal College of Midwives (RCM), is unusual among commentators in linking televised birth to the wider social context:

> Midwives around the world talk about the way the media is spreading fear of birth, but actually television and the media also reflect our culture's norms and views on birth, and the defining emotional response to birth in our culture seems to be fear. (Page 2013)

Research from media and communications as well as cultural studies has cautioned against attempts to prove causal links between media representations and audience behaviour, and called for a move beyond the 'media effects' model. The 'media effects' model is limited in so far as it positions the audience as passive and the onus of social problems is placed solely in the realm of media rather than looking to broader sociocultural structures and organisations that engender problems (see, e.g., Gauntlett 2005 [1995]). These arguments are pertinent to how we engage with televised childbirth, as the quotation from Page (above) suggests. The alternative is to take heed of recent audience reception studies that look to more complex, multifarious and negotiated ways in which people make meaning through and with television, situating engagement with television as a social process entrenched in specific societal landscapes (e.g., Skeggs and Wood 2012).

Representations of the Midwifery Profession

Midwives are charged with providing care that is evidence based (Nursing and Midwifery Council 2012), respectful and includes women in consideration of options and decision-making; this includes care during labour (National Collaborating Centre for Women's and Children's Health 2014). The extent to which this type of care is made visible through reality television requires consideration. Whether the autonomy of the midwives' role is clearly depicted in *OBEM* is open to question, as is whether those providing midwifery care are clearly differentiated from other professional (nursing) and non-professional roles (maternity care assistants). Little is shown of the 'watching and waiting' process that is a key component of midwifery work (Clifft-Matthews 2010).

Commentaries from the birth community suggest that *OBEM 'does not always portray midwives in the most sympathetic light'* (Garrod 2012). Hall sums up what is at stake:

> It matters on many levels what the public think of the profession...undermining the credibility of professional campaigns may make it harder for midwives to push through midwifery-led models of care in the face of evidence...On a more personal level, we all know the importance of building trust with women and their families. (Hall 2012)

Such concerns are not uniquely related to reality television. Kline has documented the ways in which fictional television in the United States represents midwives as stern and unsympathetic characters whose activities of work are 'trivialised and denigrated' (Kline 2010: 63); the effect is not only to ridicule the figure of the midwife but to discredit midwifery-led care and maintain the dominance of the medical model (Kline 1997, 2010). In the context of *OBEM*, two key issues of concern emerge from the commentaries. Firstly, the representation of poor practice; and secondly, the tendency to show midwives drinking tea and eating cake. The two are interconnected.

Commentators draw attention to representations of midwives as uncaring and unprofessional (e.g., Boden 2015). One key issue is the extent to which women appear to be left for long periods during labour without a midwife present. Barker (2012) observes that this portrayal of current NHS maternity services raises concerns among women. Virginia Howes started a Facebook group to highlight practice shown on *OBEM* that is 'not evidence based or woman-centred':

> '... if this really is how birth is in maternity units', she adds, 'then we should be ashamed as a profession'. (Howes, cited in Hill 2015)

However, these claims stand in contrast to a few voices—writing implicitly in response to wide-spread professional condemnation—who suggest that the show has the potential to impact *positively* on public perceptions of the profession. These defences are usually written by midwives who have participated in the show:

> ... we are proud of our profession and our service...the roles we play are not always well understood by the uninitiated...and this was a chance to show what we do. (Rogers and Dore 2010)

> I am very proud that I could demonstrate my passion for midwifery to the public. (Seddon n.d.)

This idea finds partial support in a rise in the number of students applying for midwifery undergraduate courses, a trend sometimes attributed to the popularity of programmes like *OBEM* (Furness 2013). If this is the case, it mirrors other professions that have been the subject of extensive representation in fiction and non-fiction television. Timmons and Nairn (2015) argue that the popularity of emergency medicine as a career can, in part, be linked to the high media profile of the specialism through programmes like *Casualty* and *24 Hours in A & E*—despite the ambivalence with which some clinicians view the series and concerns about how realistically their role is portrayed. Whilst increases in student applications suggests positive interpretations of television representations, at least among those considering a career in midwifery, the extent to which the programmes educate the wider public about the role and responsibilities of the midwife remains unclear.

The omnipresence of tea and cake in representations of midwives may seem trivial but it is singled out by commentators as particularly problematic:

> ... although there are parts of the programme that don't always show midwifery very accurately (we do not have that much tea and cake!). (Seddon n.d.)

> ...it may even prompt the question: are midwives always leaving couples on their own during labour, so they can pop out for a cup of tea and a natter? (The Royal College of Midwives 2012)

These concerns refer to the depiction of midwives in *OBEM* as workers who spend a substantial time engaging in humdrum chat in the staffroom. In the narrative construction of each episode, these moments provide opportunities for the audience to get to know the midwives, offering a comforting pseudo-community in a historical moment that is marked by economic insecurity, political instability and healthcare crisis (De Benedictis and Gill 2016; Hamad 2016). Such representations of healthcare workers offer comfort in times of societal uncertainty and have occurred in other historical moments (see Dovey 2000). Nevertheless, this representation of midwives as having time to sit and talk is at odds with commentators' experiences of midwifery, and stands in stark contrast to the workplace reality in the context of austerity measures, staffing cuts, long hours and work-related stress.

Entertainment or Education?

Implicit within many commentaries is the thorny question of whether *OBEM* is entertainment or education. The uncertainty of which category it belongs in may make it difficult to know by which standards it should be evaluated. However, it is deemed—within the discourse explored here—problematic as an exemplar of either category.

Whether or not the subjective experience of watching *OBEM* is entertaining, birth—so the argument goes—should not be presented for consumption as entertainment: 'How have we come to be part of a society where one of the great life transitions is seen as entertainment?' (Garrod 2012).

Some academics have argued that bringing labour and birth into the public domain has radical potential by virtue of resisting social norms of concealing the maternal body; however, the content of public representations are often problematic or conservative (Longhurst 2009). In contrast, there is a theme within the commentary pieces examined here that suggests that the broadcasting of childbirth on television per se threatens the sanctity of childbirth and signals a broader decay of societal values. Birth is presented as a drama, making an event that was previously special and reserved for the parents into one that is public, commonplace and lacking mystery (Stuthridge 2014).

However, rhetorical juxtaposition of entertainment and education, particularly in relation to bodies and health, is not unique to televised birth. Similar rhetorical devices have characterised responses to public autopsies (Miah 2004) and commercial ultrasound (Simonsen et al. 2008). In these debates 'entertainment' is used as a derogatory term by those with professional expertise to delegitimise certain cultural products. This is not to say that legitimate concerns do not exist, only that the discourse around 'entertainment' carries particular connotations and can be mobilised for strategic purposes but risks not taking women's pleasure in certain cultural products seriously (Roberts 2012). Yet public health initiatives that seek to use popular media to increase the reach and effectiveness of public-health messages (Vaughan et al. 2000; Asbeek Brusse et al. 2015) call into question whether entertainment and education are necessarily mutually exclusive.

The placement of female pain in the domain of entertainment is particularly problematic according to Boden of the campaign group Association for Improvements in the Maternity Services: 'Women's pain is trivialised as prime time viewing while people eat their tea' (Boden 2015).

De Benedictis (2017) has previously argued that *OBEM* positions viewers to react to an 'emotional rollercoaster of birth' through multiple registers of pain, joy and sentimentality. However, Boden singles out the depiction of pain as particularly problematic in the realm of 'entertainment'. Other commentators in the birth community have also made the point that childbirth and pain are sensationalised to titillate and draw in viewers, exploiting women for commercial purposes. This is a point that is mirrored in some gender studies literature. O'Brien Hill argues that *OBEM* 'makes a spectacle of the female body in pain, and part of that spectacle stems from focussing on how the expectant mother is perceived to be coping (or failing to cope) with that pain' (O'Brien Hill 2014: 192). The spectacle of emotional, and sometimes physical, pain is not unusual to the genre of reality television

(Aslama and Pantti 2006; Banet-Weiser and Portwood-Stacer 2006). There is, however, something significant about childbirth pain; it is positioned as the ultimate form of gendered pain that underlines women's potential to give birth. It is positioned outside of Western norms of the (male) body and subjectivity (see, e.g. Tyler 2000) and as such is both fascinating and unusual. Boden has strikingly termed such representations of pain in birth as 'birthporn' (Boden 2015). This reflects rhetoric in the wider literature around reality television. O'Brien Hill (2014) too argues that 'scenes of women in pain during labour are graphic, intimate and almost pornographic for the level of objectification of the body' (O'Brien Hill 2014: 192). Beyond the context of birth, Jensen (2014) explores a recent upsurge of factual welfare programming (such as *Benefit Street*) that media commentators have termed 'poverty porn' due to the sensationalising of those in poverty to create a form of 'political diversionary entertainment' (Jensen 2014: unpaginated). Commentators draw on the moral values associated with pornography in society in order to further their critiques of *OBEM* as inappropriate within the category of entertainment.

'Education' is positioned in opposition to 'entertainment', as the other category into which the programme could belong. However, this too is controversial. Commentators recognise a dearth of antenatal education and argue that this leaves *OBEM* with the task of educating women, whether or not this is the programme makers' intention. Once televised birth is cast as education, it is assessed and found wanting:

> … it's unfortunate that TV is our main source of education on something so important. (Brett 2015)
>
> … it's not put out there as an educational programme but people sometimes take what they see on TV as gospel truth. (Chamberlain 2016)

In common with other programmes within the reality television genre, *OBEM* is generically hybrid (Holmes and Jermyn 2004); it amalgamates filmic conventions from a multitude of television genres, such as documentary, soap and melodrama. In our view, the show implicitly positions itself as unmediated and educational, largely through the apparent neutrality of fixed-rig cameras being placed within 'real' hospitals, 'reflecting' 'real' childbirth events (De Benedictis 2017) while the spotlight on the intimate stories of those featured in the show simultaneously positions the programme as melodrama. This melding of conventions blurs the lines around traditional categories of genre and therefore commentators grapple over what the intent of the programme is, within the framework of broader societal discourses about television (see above)—to educate or to entertain—often with an implicit assumption that no broadcast can do both. Similarly, viewers tend to be cast in the birth community commentary as 'cultural dupes' (Adorno 2005), there is an assumption above that viewers are unable to decipher this precarious terrain of education or entertainment as they take 'what they see on TV as gospel truth', perhaps precisely because other sources of information and preparation for birth are scarce.

These issues of genre and definition are more than arguments over terminology, but rather attest to central, moral debates that have circulated for some time around reality television (Holmes and Jermyn 2004). Skeggs and Wood (2012) argue that underpinning these types of debates are fears around 'accepted notions of a "proper" public culture in liberal democracies'; the documentary has a long history of claiming to inform publics through art and the rise of reality television threatens these ideas through claims to represent reality for entertainment (although of course documentary is also constructed and also has a precarious relationship to notions of truth, albeit with different goals) (Skeggs and Wood 2012: 22). Therefore, Skeggs and Wood argue, the debates circulating around reality television are a way to create hierarchies of cultural value. Criticism of reality television from within the birth community risks falling into similar hierarchical thinking in which (actual or imagined) alternative representations of birth may be considered more valuable or effective with insufficient self-reflection on the equally constructed nature of alternatives and the values contained within them. This brings us to the question of the relationship between representation and external reality.

But Is It 'Real'?

Reality television makes strong claims to be 'real', but challenges to these claims have always been part of the genre (Biressi and Nunn 2005). Commentators from the birth community claim that the show is unrealistic:

> … show doesn't depict what labour and birth is really like for most women. (Leachman cited in Brett 2015)

TV labours are heavily edited to give a strong focus on unusual and dramatic moments and events, which do make good TV viewing but which give a distorted picture of what birth is actually like. (Garrod 2012)

The consequences of this claim are usually left unsaid. Perhaps challenging the realism of *reality* TV would seem sufficient to undermine its authority, but the history of the genre would suggest otherwise. Claims of staged performances and calculated editing have followed the format since its inception. In the context of birth the question of realism is entangled with the other themes of this chapter, with issues of birth education and fear of birth.

Claims that cultural representations are not 'real' are always problematic, relying as they do on a positivist paradigm in which reality is singular, immutable and knowable and representations can be judged to more or less closely resemble the truth. 'Truth' can be mobilised as a moral term that is often equated with a specific community's worldview (McKee 2003). *OBEM*—despite its nine series—provides only a partial representation of birth and we are sympathetic to the idea that a view of birth in line with midwifery philosophy would be a welcome addition yet mindful that this too would merely be another partial representation. Understandings, expectations and experiences of childbirth are shaped by multiple discourses, whether these are medical discourses of birth as risky and needing intervention or discourses of natural birth (Malacrida and Boulton 2014) or indeed gendered discourses of shame and birth (Lylerly 2006).

This is not to say that anything goes in representations of birth or that representations do not have real-world consequences. However, rather than asking whether *OBEM* is 'real', we might ask how birth is represented in this specific instance, who and what is present/absent in this representation and what values and assumptions underlie the construction of the show. Representations can be read in dialogue with the politics of birth in which—at least in large proportions of the global north—the obstetric model dominates and birth is culturally understood as 'risky business' (Rothman 2014). These epistemological issues also speak to questions of strategy in responding to televisual representations or intervening in popular culture. They lead to different approaches whether that is to prevent televisual depiction of birth, to provide more diversity in representations or indeed to promote media literacy.

Conclusions

Opinion pieces and commentaries written by authors from within what we have termed the 'birth community' raise vital questions about the impact of televised childbirth on women's experiences and on wider birth culture. Representations matter. However, some of the claims examined here—that *OBEM* increases fear of birth, that it damages the profession of midwifery—need a stronger empirical basis if they are to be supported. We have suggested some avenues for further research and encourage other researchers to also take up the task of examining the effects of television in the empirical domain.

If we believe that televised birth is harmful to women, then the ultimate aim must be to intervene in popular culture. *The* perfect representation of birth is unachievable but an interdisciplinary approach may offer a way forward. Central to this endeavour is conceptual clarity informed by the most up-to-date theoretical insights about the role of television in society and the mechanisms by which an impact on lived experiences might arise. Equally important is further empirical work that seeks evidence of how childbearing women, their family and friends, from across the spectrum of society, engage with televised birth in the context of their embodied lives and whether or what impact this has on issues such as preparation for birth, fear of birth, birth choices and birth experiences. We believe that interdisciplinary collaboration, in partnership with the birth community, is essential to achieving this.

Editors Note: This chapter has focused on critical responses to representations of midwifery, maternity care and childbearing women on television.

References

Adams, S.S., M. Eberhard-Gran, and A. Eskild. 2012. Fear of childbirth and duration of labour: A study of 2206 women with intended vaginal delivery. *BJOG* 119 (10): 1238–1246.

Adorno, T. 2005. Culture industry reconsidered. In *Popular culture: A reader*, ed. R. Guins and O.Z. Cruz, 103–108. London: Sage.

Asbeek Brusse, E.D., M.L. Fransen, and E.G. Smit. 2015. Educational storylines in entertainment television: Audience reactions toward persuasive strategies in medical dramas. *Journal of Health Communication* 20 (4): 396–405.

Aslama, M., and M. Pantti. 2006. Talking alone: Reality TV, emotions and authenticity. *European Journal of Cultural Studies* 9 (2): 167–184.

Banet-Weiser, S., and L. Portwood-Stacer. 2006. 'I just want to be me again!': Beauty pageants, reality television and post-feminism. *Feminist Theory* 7 (2): 255–272.

Barker, K. 2012. Is midwifery still a labour of love? *British Journal of Midwifery* 20 (5): 378.

Biressi, A., and H. Nunn. 2005. *Reality TV: Realism and revelation*. New York: Wallflower Press.

Boden, G. 2015. Childbirth as entertainment. *Association for Improvements in the Maternity Services (AIMS)* 24 (4). http://www.aims.org.uk/?Journal/Vol24No4/birthAsEntertainment.htm.

Brett, M. 2015. Petition to ban One Born Every Minute. Retrieved October 25, 2016, from http://theworkingparent.com/petition-to-ban-one-born-every-minute/.

Chamberlain, Z. 2016. One Born Every Minute should be banned because it scares pregnant women, says therapist. Retrieved October 25, 2016, from http://www.mirror.co.uk/news/uk-news/one-born-every-minute-should-7164824.

Clifft-Matthews, V. 2010. Vaginal birth as a rite of passage. *British Journal of Midwifery* 18 (3): 140.

De Benedictis, S. 2017. Watching One Born Every Minute: Negotiating the terms of the 'good birth'. In *Television for women*, ed. R. Mosely, H. Wheatley, and H. Wood, 110–127. Oxon: Routledge.

De Benedictis, S., and R. Gill. 2016. Austerity neoliberalism: A new discursive formation. Retrieved November 10, 2016, from https://www.opendemocracy.net/uk/austerity-media/sara-de-benedictis-rosalind-gill/austerity-neoliberalism-new-discursive-formation.

Dovey, J. 2000. *Freakshow: First person media and factual television*. London: Pluto Press.

Fenwick, J., J. Toohill, D.K. Creedy, J. Smith, and J. Gamble. 2015. Sources, responses and moderators of childbirth fear in Australian women: A qualitative investigation. *Midwifery* 31 (1): 239–246.

Furness, H. 2013. Call the Midwife sparks surge in student applications. Retrieved October 25, 2016, from http://www.telegraph.co.uk/culture/tvandradio/bbc/9794531/CalltheMidwifesparkssurgeinstudentapplications.html.

Garrod, D. 2012. Birth as entertainment: What are the wider effects? *British Journal of Midwifery* 20 (2): 81.

Gauntlett, D. 2005 [1995]. *Moving experiences: Understanding television's influences and effects*. Eastleigh: John Libbey.

Gill, R. 2007. *Gender and the media*. Cambridge: Polity Press.

Greer, J., A. Lazenbatt, and L. Dunne. 2014. 'Fear of childbirth' and ways of coping for pregnant women and their partners during the birthing process: A salutogenic analysis. *Evidence Based Midwifery* 12 (3): 95–100.

Hall, A. 2012. Maintaining trust in the profession. *British Journal of Midwifery* 20 (2): 80.
Hamad, H. 2016. Contemporary medical television and crisis in the NHS. *Critical Studies in Television: The International Journal of Television Studies* 11 (2): 136–150.
Hill, M. 2015. Love birth? You probably hate One Born Every Minute? Retrieved October 25, 2016, from http://www.positivebirthmovement.org/pbm-blog/love-birth-you-probably-hate-one-born-every-minute.
Holmes, S., and D. Jermyn. 2004. *Understanding reality television*. London: Routledge.
Jensen, T. 2014. Welfare commonsense, poverty porn and doxosophy. *Sociological Research Online* 19 (3): no pagination.
Kline, K.N. 1997. Midwife attended births in prime-time television: Craziness, controlling bitches, and ultimate capitulation. *Women and Language* 30 (1): 20–29.
Kline, K.N. 2010. Poking fun at midwifery on prime-time television: The rhetorical implications of burlesque frames in humorous shows. *Women and Language* 33 (1): 53–71.
Laursen, M., C. Johansen, and M. Hedegaard. 2009. Fear of childbirth and risk for birth complications in nulliparous women in the Danish National Birth Cohort. *BJOG* 116 (10): 1350–1355.
Leachman, A. 2015. The problem with One Born Every Minute. Retrieved October 25, 2016, from http://www.fearfreechildbirth.com/blog/one-born-every-minute/.
Longhurst, R. 2009. YouTube: A new space for birth? *Feminist Review* 93: 46–63.
Lothian, J.A., and A. Grauer. 2003. "Reality" birth: Marketing fear to childbearing women. *The Journal of Perinatal Education* 12 (2): vi–viii.
Luce, A., M. Cash, V. Hundley, H. Cheyne, E. van Teijlingen, and C. Angell. 2016. "Is it realistic?" The portrayal of pregnancy and childbirth in the media. *BMC Pregnancy and Childbirth* 16 (1): 1–10.
Lylerly, A.D. 2006. Shame, gender, birth. *Hypatia* 21 (1): 101–118.
Malacrida, C., and T. Boulton. 2014. The best laid plans? Women's choices, expectations and experiences in childbirth. *Health (London)* 18 (1): 41–59.
McKee, A. 2003. *Textual analysis: A beginner's guide*. London: Sage.
Miah, A. 2004. The public autopsy: Somewhere between art, education, and entertainment. *Journal of Medical Ethics* 30 (6): 576–579.
Munro, S., J. Kornelsen, and E. Hutton. 2009. Decision making in patient-initiated elective cesarean delivery: The influence of birth stories. *Journal of Midwifery & Women's Health* 54 (5): 373–379.
National Collaborating Centre for Women's and Children's Health. 2014. Version 2. Intrapartum Care Clinical Guideline 190 December 2014.

Nursing and Midwifery Council. 2012. Midwives rules and standards 2012. www.nmc.org.uk. NMC. 2016.

O'Brien Hill, G.E. 2014. The older mother in One Born Every Minute. In *Ageing, popular culture and contemporary feminism: Harleys and hormones*, ed. I. Whelehan and J. Gwynne, 187–202. Basingstoke: Palgrave Macmillan.

Page, L. 2013. Birth in the bright lights. *British Journal of Midwifery* 21 (4): 234.

Richens, Y., C. Hindley, and T. Lavender. 2015. A national online survey of UK maternity unit service provision for women with fear of birth. *British Journal of Midwifery* 23 (8): 574–579.

Roberts, J. 2012. *The visualised foetus: A cultural and political analysis of ultrasound imagery*. Farnham: Ashgate Publishing Limited.

Rogers, J., and M. Dore. 2010. One Born Every Minute... how it was for us. Retrieved October 25, 2016, from https://www.rcm.org.uk/news-views-and-analysis/analysis/one-born-every-minute-how-it-was-for-us.

Rothman, B.K. 2014. Pregnancy, birth and risk: An introduction. *Health, Risk & Society* 16 (1): 1–6.

Seddon, E. (n.d.). When I was on One Born Every Minute.... Retrieved October 25, 2016, from http://www.midwifecareer.com/when-i-was-on-one-born-every-minute/.

Simonsen, S.E., D.W. Branch, and N.C. Rose. 2008. The complexity of fetal imaging: Reconciling clinical care with patient entertainment. *Obstetrics and Gynecology* 112 (6): 1351–1354.

Skeggs, B., and H. Wood. 2012. *Reacting to reality television: Performance, audience and value*. Abingdon: Routledge.

Stuthridge, T. 2014. The midwife blog: Birth and social technology. Retrieved October 25, 2016, from https://www.midirs.org/midwife-blog-june/.

The Royal College of Midwives. 2012. Behind the scenes. Retrieved October 25, 2016, from https://www.rcm.org.uk/news-views-and-analysis/analysis/behind-the-scenes.

Thomson, G., K. Stoll, S. Downe, and W.A. Hall. 2017. Negative impressions of childbirth in a North-West England student population. *Journal of Psychosomatic Obstetrics & Gynecology* 38 (1): 37–44.

Timmons, S., and S. Nairn. 2015. The development of the specialism of emergency medicine: Media and cultural influences. *Health (London)* 19 (1): 3–16.

Tyler, I. 2000. Reframing pregnant embodiment. In *Transformations: Thinking through feminism*, ed. S. Ahmed, J. Kilby, C. Lury, M. McNeil, and B. Skeggs, 288–302. London: Routledge.

Vaughan, W., M. Everett, A. Rogers, M. Singhal Ramadhan, and P. Swalehe. 2000. Entertainment-education and HIV/AIDS prevention: A field experiment in Tanzania. *Journal of Health Communication* 5 (suppl. 1): 81–100.

CHAPTER 3

Birth Stories in British Newspapers: Why Midwives Must Speak up

Emily Maclean

Abstract A free press is held to be a benchmark of healthy society—but this chapter explores how British newspapers may contribute to adverse birth outcomes. Social theory about news-making suggests that the experience of having a baby has emotive human interest, and editors tend to favour those which are unusual. Hence the deliveries which make it into print are out-of-the-ordinary, often frightening and likely to distort readers' risk perceptions. Such a dynamic may be a factor in increased rates of caesarean section, which has been associated with fearful future mothers, medicalised care and interventionist policymakers. This prompts a call for midwives to engage with journalists in order to represent vaginal birth as a normal bodily function which has benefits for both mother and baby. Giving interviews is acknowledged to be an intimidating prospect for most clinicians; hence high-quality media training is essential. Maclean concludes by giving insights about how a newsroom works, and suggests that if editors are given sufficiently interesting material, they may find space for more normal birth stories. There is no expectation for newspapers to stop holding clinicians to account or

E. Maclean (✉)
London School of Hygiene and Tropical Medicine, London, UK
e-mail: emilyjanemaclean@gmail.com

© The Author(s) 2017
A. Luce et al. (eds.), *Midwifery, Childbirth and the Media*,
DOI 10.1007/978-3-319-63513-2_3

to 'change' the media. Rather, advocates of normal birth might better understand how news-making works, so as to help meet the aforementioned criteria for a good story. Maclean concedes that even as a former journalist, it is stressful being a midwife who grants media requests. But her experience of such exposure suggests this is an opportunity not to be wasted.

Keywords Representations · Newspapers · Birth · Midwives Extreme event

INTRODUCTION

Like it or loathe it, a free press is part of the United Kingdom's national fabric. Newspaper articles can help maintain National Health Service (NHS) standards by calling authorities to account, highlighting poor practice and informing readers on issues that underpin their well-being (Allan 2010; Conboy 2011; Leveson 2012). However, newspapers also need to make money and this is not always good for our health (Tulloch and Lupton 2003). The NHS webpage *Behind the Headlines*, which seeks to 'give the facts without the fiction', shows that tales which grab our attention may not be wholly representative of the situation at hand (NHS Choices 2016). This is certainly true of birth, which is usually a pivotal family moment, but not a news event. The rare occasions that do make it into print often share one common feature: they are out of the ordinary. A landmark study into the process of newsmaking identified several factors that increase the odds an incident will be reported (Galtung and Ruge 1965). These included 'human interest' and a 'culturally familiar' situation, two boxes both ticked by even the most ordinary of birth stories (Harcup and O'Neill 2001). Yet a third factor was an element of the 'unexpected or rare'—something which distinguishes most women's experiences from those which sell newspapers. Hence, the headline 'Woman has Straightforward Labour and Healthy Baby' would not get published. Consequently, the information available in the powerful national press inevitably gives a non-representative view of what birth is like—both for expectant mothers and other stakeholders, including policy makers. It is likely to emphasise the unusual, failing to reflect the fact that 60% of mothers in England have a spontaneous vaginal birth, are not celebrities, and do not have babies on trains or in car parks; moreover, majority receive adequate care (Cumberledge 2016; NHS 2016).

This chapter examines how the experience of giving birth is portrayed in the UK national newspapers, using articles from a review outlined below. It confirms the suspicion that childbirth is invariably represented as an extreme event, with powerful messages that may distort the risk perception of future mothers. The analysis considers how different story 'frames' (e.g., horror, celebrity, and debate) each distance women from normal birth in a variety of ways (Allan 2010). The discussion notes clinical evidence that confirms birth is a normal physiological event and labour is often neither dramatic nor high risk (Renfrew et al. 2014). It considers the potential public health impact of such media reports, including whether fear of birth may be rising across society, perhaps contributing to rising rates of caesarean section (NHS 2016). The noise created by tabloid and broadsheet headlines is also compared.

Insights from the author's previous career in journalism demystify how information reaches the public domain and supports a case for midwives, as advocates for normal birth, to engage more proactively with the media. Such exposure can be daunting. Yet the author's recent experience representing midwives in newspapers and on TV has shown that journalists and their audiences do not expect perfection, and it pays to communicate.

METHODS

There was limited evidence on the UK newspaper coverage of birth until the author performed a newspaper review of reports published in national titles, including daily and Sunday editions of the *Evening Standard, Express, The Guardian, Independent, Mail, Metro, Mirror, Sun, The Daily Telegraph* and *The Times* (Maclean 2014a). This chapter draws new insights from this study, which involved thematic analysis of women's stories published over a 12-month period (December 2011–November 2012). A search of the Newspaper Licensing Agency database, using the terms 'My and Birth and Midwife', yielded 198 first-person accounts about the experience of having a vaginal birth. The legitimacy or trustworthiness of reports played no part in the analysis; the purpose was to assess what a story said, rather than how or why it had been constructed. Grounded Theory informed the analysis, which led to 61 emergent codes, including fear, ordeal, pain, effective staff, malicious or poor care, intervention, humour, positive pain, relief, no choice, infection, no pain and mother's instinct.

Headlines

The interest now is the impression given by such stories' headlines. Arguably these epitomise the journalistic act of pinpointing drama further still, as attention-grabbing, active phrases compete for the reader's interest and encapsulate the 'top line' of a story (Zelizer and Allan 2010). In emphasising a report's shock factor, they may be more likely to stick in people's memory (Ecker et al. 2014). The content for review was then narrowed down further to headlines containing first-person statements, such as 'Midwife infected me', a story explored below. Direct quotes have been identified as having a significant impact on readers, inspiring trust, and often seeming closer to events (Gibson and Zillmann 1993; Sundar 1998; Zelizer 1989). Mothers telling stories 'in their own words' may also function as 'peer-reports' (shared experience between individuals in similar situations), which are known to exert an influence on women when they are making decisions about place of birth (Coxon et al. 2014).

LITERATURE REVIEW

One UK-based study cited a mid-market article entitled 'Are you too posh to push?' exploring the cultural climate around caesarean delivery on maternal request (Kingdon 2009). The double-page feature in the *Daily Mail* framed it as a class issue, suggesting a lifestyle of 'convenience pregnancy' might be emerging, with the implication that abdominal surgery was considered by some to be preferable to vaginal delivery (Moorhead 1999). Subsequently, Kingdon gave a broad assessment of how British newspapers described the two modes of birth, noting that neither was portrayed 'particularly positively' (2009). Beyond the UK, analysis of coverage in Australian daily, *The Age* found 'risk' to be a dominant issue (McIntyre et al. 2011). A study into women's-magazine culture in the United States found labour described as a 'marathon', requiring abdominal muscle training (Dworkin and Wachs 2004). Subsequently, an article about how birth is reflected in online news found that midwives were depicted as inferior to obstetricians (Dahlen and Homer 2012). Several critiques have incorporated print publications into analyses of broadcast media, with a notable UK example suggesting that an absence of normal birth on television might be perpetuating the medicalisation of childbirth (Luce et al. 2016). Research in Australia linked coverage of childbirth issues to higher rates of elective caesarean (Robson et al. 2008). Meanwhile, women's choice of place of birth (midwife- or obstetric-led unit, or at home) seems prompted by factors including media reports and a 'culture of fatalism' that is associated with a risk-averse press (Coxon et al. 2014; Houghton et al. 2008). Meanwhile, global midwifery figures have questioned the impact of news reports on public consciousness about maternity issues, and on women's health policy-making (Bick 2010; Dahlen 2010; Young et al. 2008).

Risk Perception

Before this chapter delves into the newspaper material itself, it is important to outline some social theory about how the press may affect women's birthing behaviour and maternity service commissioners' allocation of resources. This also foregrounds a challenge to midwives to summon the confidence and determination to find ways of making the case for straightforward vaginal birth interesting to today's media.

Newspapers have been identified as drivers of what some term 'risk society' (Beck 1992). In such a culture, the desire to minimise the chance of adverse events outweighs other priorities (e.g. personal choice). The media and other social elites breed a widespread belief that interventions and regulations are needed in order for life to run safely. Applied to birth, hospital is seen as a necessary way of regaining control over nature, almost a means to 'save' women from labour and birth (Foucault 1976; Scamell 2014). The distortion of risk is exemplified by a *Guardian* headline 'My granny delivered my baby'. While tens of thousands of people will have read this, relatively few will have accessed an academic survey report that showed only 0.5% of births in the UK occur without a practitioner present (NPEU 2010). This could prompt women to expect panic and danger from birth, which leads some to attend hospital earlier in labour (Nolan 2009). Being in a facility longer increases another kind of risk: 'the cascade of intervention' that may include being strapped to a foetal heart monitor, needing a synthetic hormone drip to boost contractions, and ending up in theatre for a caesarean section (Janssen and Desmarais 2013; Rossignol et al. 2014). While obstetric support is central to modern maternity care, saving lives and improving outcomes, the risk profile of most women is lower than media messages suggest.

Of course women and other stakeholders critique the extent to which press coverage reflects real life; it has long been theorised that any audience has its own filter (Lacey 2002). Yet emotive stories can have an impact on an individual's perceptions and unconscious bias (Loewenstein et al. 2001). An NHS services commissioner might be moved disproportionately by this kind of story, especially if several come in quick succession, creating a feeling of public consensus on the topic (Buse et al. 2012). Indeed, political anxiety about managing birth has prompted societies to increase routine medical intervention into what is essentially a normal female bodily function (Donnison 1977).

Fear of Birth

Pregnant women often feel vulnerable, and there is plenty of scope for the headlines explored below to create implicit meanings that are frightening (Rich and Zaragoza 2016). This is of concern, as fear of birth has been attributed to a range of adverse reproductive outcomes, including phobia of becoming pregnant (Hofberg and Ward 2004), seeking abortion (Larsson et al. 2002), elective caesarean section (Fenwick et al. 2009; Haines et al. 2011), emergency caesarean section (Ryding et al. 1998), mental health problems (Rouhe et al. 2011) and prolonged labour (Johnson and Slade 2003; Adams et al. 2012). Leading proponents of normal birth have documented how fear inhibits the natural hormonal processes which allow most women to give birth naturally (Dick-Read 2004; Odent 2013). Midwives are well-placed to alleviate women's fears through an antenatal one-to-one discussion about what labour can feel like, how it usually works and what clinical processes might be involved (Fenwick et al. 2015). Here it is argued that midwives should extend the conversation beyond individual consultations and calm nerves on a wider scale by informing newspaper stories through quotes and off-record briefings. Admittedly, such exposure is itself not without risk—as discussed later.

Public Health

The public health implications of the articles explored here are significant, not least because greater intervention in labour brings greater cost (Tracy and Tracy 2003). Medicalising birth does not improve outcomes, as large-scale research on the benefits of midwifery care for low-risk women has confirmed (Renfrew et al. 2014). Two studies of recent years have made waves in academic circles and influenced clinical guidelines—promoting midwife-led birth, often at home, and continuity of care (Brocklehurst et al. 2011; NICE 2014; Sandall et al. 2016). But personal experience indicates that women often seem surprised by this kind of information. The message is not getting through to 'their' media. Such a situation may rob them of informed choice and the opportunity to demand appropriate services (Fenwick et al. 2015).

Real Life and Normal Birth: Not on the Same Page

The excerpts below distance normal women from the prospect of having a baby calmly and naturally, in three ways. First, they may show ordinary individuals having out-of-the ordinary experiences, including cruel or dangerous midwives, stillbirth, tokophobia (a disorder: the extreme fear of birth), and complications, including pre-eclampsia. Second, headlines might frame a straightforward vaginal birth (be it at home, or very quickly) as somehow freaky. Third, many successful vaginal birth stories often belong to celebrities, on a pedestal as something to aspire to, but in a luxury or superhuman context that may be out of reach. Meanwhile, it is noted that celebrity horror stories, of which there are several, are likely to stick in people's minds (Farrell 2013).

AVERAGE WOMEN, WORSE-THAN-AVERAGE STORIES

Malicious, Dangerous Midwives

Several newspapers depict midwives as malevolent figures, who cause harm by negligence, incompetence or wilful wrong-doing. Allegations include one in the *Evening Standard*: 'Midwife simply laughed at my torment over stillborn baby'. This tells how a birth brought not only tragedy but also cruel treatment at the hands of NHS staff. Meanwhile, a headline in the *Sunday Express* heralds how midwives had failed to heed a mother's warnings about her baby's condition: 'I trusted the midwives... If they'd listened to me, my angel would still be alive'. The same publication has a story entitled 'Don't call the midwife, she'll shout at me!' The recent National Maternity Review lamented that some women do receive inexcusably poor care; it is essential that newspapers raise such issues (Cumberledge 2016). But the author also noted how investigations identified midwives who were kind and skilled. However, these benign characteristics do not fire the imagination (and inspire headlines) in the way a wicked woman can (Allan 2010). It is an issue which has long frustrated feminists (Ehrenreich and English 2010).

Meanwhile, the *Daily Mail* tells of a midwife who was both dangerous and diseased: 'Midwife infected me with hepatitis C as I was giving birth'. As with the headlines above, this one carries active, personal language; it shocks. If read by a pregnant woman, it has a high chance of creating antenatal anxiety. NHS midwives are routinely screened for infectious diseases, but this individual was apparently missed. So despite the fact that the average individual stands a greater probability of being harmed while going about their everyday life, the article plants a seed of fear that this could happen to you (Beck 1992).

Losing a Baby

Several headlines blame staff for the deaths of babies, including one in the *Times*: 'Friends saw my baby wasn't growing—midwives didn't'. Meanwhile, a *Sunday Times* article exemplifies how a headline might distort the risk perception of not only the birthing mother, but also those who commission her care. The report is headed, '"My baby's dead, isn't she, nurse?" Girl's Death in a Midwife Unit Has Fuelled the Row Over Centres Not Staffed by Obstetricians'. It involves a legal ruling that a baby died because there were no doctors in the freestanding midwife-led unit where a 35-year-old woman was in labour. The baby died six hours after being born, and an inquest ruled that the mother should have been referred to an obstetric-led facility due to complications towards the end of her pregnancy. The incident merits reporting on grounds of public interest, and of course, no firm conclusion can be drawn as to how the piece might affect readers' perceptions of midwifery care. Yet it is reasonable to suggest that perceptions could be skewed negatively (Tulloch and Lupton 2003). The article has gravitas, written in the conservative tone of a broadsheet, which gives a sense of measured reason. Yet the colloquial headline is stomach-churning. This could affect the birthplace choices of women, and also their trusted friends and family—important sounding boards for expectant mothers (Coxon et al. 2014). We live in a litigious age where stories like this matter, because public image matters (Scamell 2014). Such a headline has the power to reinforce clinicians' tendency to intervene in labour and birth, despite evidence that this does not necessarily improve maternal or child health (Cheng et al. 2014). Further up the hierarchy, a service commissioner is unlikely to be drawn towards this model of care when reading a grieving mother says: 'I hope women are better informed about the dangers, the real, massive risks of delivering in a midwife-led unit. I think stand-alone midwife-led units should provide antenatal care and postnatal care but they should not be used for deliveries' (Templeton 2012). A health minister may also navigate a normative, biomedical path away from such a birth environment, given that 'the political sphere can only ignore published opinion at the risk of losing votes' (Beck 1992). Of course, such professionals consult a range of materials when planning, but an emotive story is disproportionately powerful for decision-makers, as 'risk-as-feelings' often predominate over cognitive assessments (Loewenstein et al. 2001).

The added visibility given to this worst-case scenario by the act of publication for 2.5 million *Sunday Times* readers will never be balanced by stories about happy, healthy births in freestanding midwifery-led units (National Readership Survey 2013). Ultimately, 'when perceived pregnancy risk is out of proportion to real risk, and when risk management procedures are applied to all pregnant women with benefit for a few, unintended and harmful consequences may result' (Jordan and Murphy 2009; p. 198). A possible upshot is the aforementioned 'cascade of intervention' (Tracy and Tracy 2003).

There are also heartbreaking headlines from women describing the sheer tragedy of losing a baby. A lottery winner tells the *Sun*, 'I'd bought my twins matching sailor outfits to leave hospital but Mason never came home'. Meanwhile, *The Mail on Sunday* gives an account of stillbirth under the headline 'Our day of tragedy—and the memories we cherish'. The piece goes on to say that the 'stillbirth rate, of 4.9 per 1000 births in 2010, is the lowest recorded'. Yet the dominant—and arguably misleading—impression is left by the headline (Ecker et al. 2014).

Medical Complications in Pregnancy

Some reports carry headlines concerning potentially fatal maternal conditions associated with pregnancy—for instance, pre-eclampsia. A *Sun* report is headed: 'My baby was dead and my organs were shutting down'. A subheading reads 'Killer Condition That Affects 30,000 Mums-To-Be Every Year'. The piece promotes senior obstetricians' concerns that services were suboptimal for 9 in 10 women who die from the condition (Neilson 2011; Shennan et al. 2012). A statistic tends to raise the impression of trustworthiness in a report—but these numbers are relatively meaningless unless we know the prevalence of fatal pre-eclampsia in pregnancy in the United Kingdom. It is not common at all; two women died from the condition during pregnancy in 2012–2014 (Knight et al. 2016). One of the obstetricians referenced in the *Sun* story has recently stated that 'pregnancy has never been safer'—but his piece in

The Lancet, calling for yet better care, did not make it into more popular publications (Shennan et al. 2017). The *Sun* headline is not wrong, but it is likely to give readers a false impression that might lead to heightened nerves in pregnancy (Scamell 2014).

The dynamic is similar for another *Sun* headline, 'Gastric bypass almost killed my baby', with warnings from a 27-year-old mother who dropped from 30 to 21 stone while pregnant. This gives the impression that birth is a traumatic and dangerous prospect after having the operation—but taking time to shed weight before trying for a baby markedly improves a woman's risk profile (Khan et al. 2013). The Royal College of Obstetricians and Gynaecologists (RCOG) says such an intervention should be a last resort, but states it is safer to be pregnant after surgery than to conceive while morbidly obese (2015). Such a piece could have been both improved and informed by a midwife voice's empathising with the (human interest) emotion of the situation, while also promoting individualised care which sees the person behind the condition. This is particularly important in cases of medical complexity, where efforts to normalise labour can improve outcomes and maternal satisfaction (Royal College of Midwives (RCM) 2012).

Elsewhere, headlines introduce more 'everyday' troubles, such as the exhaustion that labour can bring. *The Guardian* has mothers writing comment pieces based on their birth experiences, one asking 'Was it so tiring first time round?' while another states: 'No birth is without risk'. In the latter mother is citing personal experiences of a traumatic labour which ended in an emergency caesarean section, in response to debates about 'free birth', where medical services are avoided. A *Daily Telegraph* first-person piece discusses 'tokophobia'—extreme fear of giving birth vaginally—with the headline, 'I Was Terrified That If I had a Baby It Would Kill Me'.

Ordinary Women, 'Freak' Stories

'Born Before Arrival'

When a baby is born quickly, the mother's natural physiology is usually working well (Dick-Read 2004). Yet several headlines imply that something is out of kilter in fast labours. *The Guardian* has the startling phrases 'My granny delivered my baby' and 'I delivered my own baby'. A midwife tells the *Mirror* 'I'm a DIY midwife' after catching her own child. Meanwhile, *People* shows a series of novelty stories called 'Oh Blimey! Births', including the case of a hypno-birthing couple who were 'Caught on the hop'. These upbeat stories merit being told. They also echo clinical evidence and demonstrate how women have the capacity to follow their bodies and give birth successfully with minimal intervention (Brocklehurst et al. 2011). However, they arguably don't 'normalise' birth, as all are treated as entertaining freak cases, something 'unexpected or rare' (Galtung and Ruge 1965). The headlines conjure almost cartoonish impressions of a grandmother crouching between her granddaughter's legs, or a birthing woman wearing a midwife's uniform. Of course, it is the job of such phrases to paint a picture in a few short words—but this leaves little room for nuance (Reah 2002). It is probable that some childbearing readers could appraise these quick-birthing peers and see them as almost unreal, as something 'other'. They are thus potentially distanced from the prospect of having a normal vaginal birth. Several of these stories involve so-called born before arrival (BBA) births—where the midwife or doctor is not yet present. A BBA is rare, affecting fewer than 1% of babies (Unterscheider et al. 2011). Yet straightforward vaginal births are common, as indicated by national statistics (NHS 2016). The 'novelty' story type thus overshadows the story of straightforward vaginal birth with a feature that makes it unusual.

Surprises and Miracles

There are also tales of surprise babies, where the birth goes well but is overshadowed by the fact that it was unexpected. 'My gorgeous little accident' was conceived despite the mother being on the contraceptive pill; and another woman says, 'I didn't know I was having a baby, until my stomach ache turned out to be labour pains'. While these stories emphasise how women can carry and have babies without even thinking about it, the headlines also associate normal birth with something out of the ordinary.

Home Birth

Despite the fact that home births are recommended for any low-risk second-time mother, newspapers often depict those women who choose to give birth out of hospital as unusual (NICE 2014). The coverage was not necessarily negative; the *Daily Mail* ran the headline 'My home birth was fast and furious, but so amazing'. This does not suggest labour is easy, but neither does it appear traumatic. This example stands out in demonstrating it is possible for a normal birth story to be interesting to a mass-market newspaper audience. Yet the *Daily Mail* also has a piece which asks the question, 'Why Would Any Woman Choose To Give Birth in Front of Her Children?' with the subheading: 'I Was in Labour While the Boys Ate Their Tea—They Kept Coming Over To Ask If The Baby Was Out Yet. In the End I Shouted: "Just Get Them Out Of Here!"' This depicts home birth as chaotic and stressful, rather than a way of increasing the chances of a normal delivery and good outcomes (Brocklehurst et al. 2011). *The Guardian* gives a different angle, reporting a mother's story of doing baking while in labour, under the header 'We love to eat Eliza's birthday cake'. This creates a sense that a vaginal birth at home can be part of the everyday, but this baking birther is every inch the domestic goddess. She borders on being one of the 'celebocracy' figures discussed below, to be admired but not emulated (Farrell 2013). Meanwhile, the *Sun* pours cold water on aspirations for an all-natural experience under the headline 'The best laid (birth) plans'. The feature includes lines like 'I wanted a hypnobirth', 'An hour after the birth I was in my own bed', and 'I was Naive about how Painful it would be'. These are not all negative, but the use of capitals emphasises scarier aspects of the latter story. Here, then, is an array of birth stories which by no means ruin the image of home birth, but neither do they make it seem particularly do-able.

Normal Birth on a Pedestal: Celebrities

The third dynamic identified in this research involves celebrities, whose stories have become a genre in themselves as the public's appetite for behind-the-scenes information grows. The production of such material does not always stem from the incident itself, but rather a mutually beneficial relationship between the publication, which sells more copies when its cover is graced by a famous face—and the individuals themselves, who often have a lifestyle, brand or product to promote (Farrell 2013). This may mean that the 'reality' the stories depict is idealised, in order to prompt followers' aspiration, and/or improve a celebrity's public image in the face of negative expose-style stories. Equally, the disclosure of a difficult experience could inspire affection or respect. This is not to claim that the people cited below were cynical in their actions, but rather to acknowledge that what appears to be a candid, intimate process of storytelling is often subject to external influences.

Celebration

Several sit-down interviews cast birth in positive light—even if it is portrayed as a feat of endurance. Olympic champion Fatima Whitbread tells the *Daily Mail*, 'My son is worth a million medals'. Case studies come from *One Born Every Minute*, with mothers commenting on what was seen on-screen, under headlines such as the *Sun's* 'Why We Gave Birth in Front of the Cameras'. The narratives mirror the programme's dynamics, pinpointing the most dramatic moments. An opera singer who was filmed with her husband (James) while having an emergency caesarean reflects on the impact her story may have had on women's perceptions. She says, 'When I suggested to James about doing the programme, it was because I wanted to show women that it's possible to have a lovely, natural, positive experience. Which is ironic really?' Meanwhile, model Penny Lancaster tells her story in the *Daily Express* under the banner 'I Was Born To Be A Mum', describing a happy memory of water birth alongside husband Rod Stewart. The glossy tone might give the impression that such a labour is unattainable for most women. Yet it also suggests that birth need not sap a woman of energy and beauty. Meanwhile, a straight-talking article was written by broadcaster Jenni Murray, who responds to a debate about epidurals with the headline in the *Daily Mail* "Get Real, Girls! Pain Is Part of Childbirth'. She narrates her own experience of normal birth, which involved being in a secluded, dark environment. Hence celebrity stories give mixed impressions of what it's like to have a baby—and at best, the effect has potential to inform rather than frighten. Yet readers may not be able to put themselves in such successful women's shoes. This may due to a social culture designed to put celebrities on a pedestal and idealise their lives (including giving birth) (Farrell 2013).

Ordeal

Several famous women have had double-page spreads devoted to traumatic vaginal births. This is likely to provoke readers' sympathy, but as noted above, it might also create anxiety for women of childbearing age and their support networks. In the *Daily Mail*, Jenny Agutter, an actress in *Call The Midwife*, says, 'My son was five weeks premature. All hell was let loose'. In the *Mail on Sunday* Michelle Heaton, a singer, says, 'I was told I might need open heart surgery...at the same time as I was having my baby'. Lesley Gilchrist, who is depicted as a 'star' in the Sun after appearing on the reality show *One Born Every Minute*, says, 'I lost my brother—eight weeks later I almost lost my little girl'. A weather forecaster describes having a premature birth, while another singer (Mylene Klass) tells the *Daily Express* of crippling pelvic girdle pain with the headline 'Having a Baby Left Me in Agony'. Celebrity stories are common 'water-cooler' topics of conversation, so these horror stories are likely to have been fixed into individual and public consciousness more firmly than they would have been had their subjects been anonymous (Farrell 2013). This could exacerbate the impact of risk aversion discussed earlier, creating a sense that vaginal birth brings trauma and agony.

Broadsheet Versus Tabloid

The sample has more tabloid than broadsheet stories with first-person titles, perhaps reflecting the tendency to give reports a sense of immediacy through direct quotation. Yet an array of articles across the spectrum carry mothers' perspectives on pain in labour. A *Daily Telegraph* writer has 'A Bone To Pick With the Birth Mother' when interviewing Sheila Kitzinger, an anthropologist who has suggested that some women could feel sexual sensations during labour and birth (2012). The journalist goes on to say, 'if a ventouse, forceps and enough postpartum stitches to update the Bayeux Tapestry counts as an orgasm, I've clearly been doing it wrong for years'. Through clever language, the notion of managing a vaginal birth well is ripped to shreds. *The Express* explores different approaches to pain management by incorporating a more diverse range of perspectives, taking a chronological look at different women's experiences through the decades. Its headlines say: 'The only men allowed were doctors', 'I was so glad to have modern pain relief', 'Having our baby at home was right for us'. Another article cites a woman saying that birth 'left me traumatised', alongside the headline 'Natural Birth Losing Out to the Epidural'. This serves to confirm that simplistic points of view are by no means the preserve of redtop (or tabloid) titles. All types of newspaper in this review have produced some balanced, informative pieces; and they are each equally capable of the other extreme. Thus readers of all socio-economic backgrounds are exposed to a variety of headlines. This in itself presents a mandate for midwives to engage with the broadest range of newspapers possible.

Media Engagement

Getting the Press to Call the Midwife

These findings prompt a repeat of previous suggestions that more engagement between midwives and the media is essential (Hundley et al. 2015; Luce et al 2016; Maclean 2014a). From 2004 to 2011, I worked as a national newspaper reporter for titles ranging from the *Daily Mirror* to the *Telegraph*. Since joining the NHS, I have found there is considerable—and often understandable—fear of giving interviews to journalists. This needs to be resolved. The tales and opinions of rankand-file midwives arguably have 'human interest' appeal, which might be exploited to occupy popular print spaces and rebalance the view of birth. The potential for personal angles about normal vaginal birth has been underscored by traction in print and broadcast media created by midwife and mother Clemmie Hooper's book *How to Grow a Baby and Push it Out* (2017). Only by embracing the kind of stories newspapers want to print—for example, tear-jerkers—can midwives find a vehicle for getting their voice heard. The line between print, broadcast and online media is disappearing, as each feeds the other—which increases the impact any single interaction may have.

Inside the Newsroom

When I was working as a reporter, I wanted to tell good stories, preferably meaningful ones. It could have been fascinating to write about 'A day in the life of a labour ward'. But getting access to such an environment felt fraught with difficulty. In a fast-paced, demanding industry, there were alternative ways of sourcing legitimate material, be they inquests, public reports or phone calls from readers who might ring in with personal stories. If a press officer had offered me 24 hours on a midwife-led unit, I would have jumped at the chance, and found a way of keeping both the NHS and my editors happy. Such information-gathering might have expanded my awareness about the process of having a baby in a low-risk setting, hopefully even prompting a piece that found human interest in this pivotal family event. Of course, women would need to consent to their story being told. But if having a vaginal birth can happen on television, for instance in the upbeat drama *Call the Midwife*, it can happen in the papers.

Inside the NHS

Now that I am on the other side of the fence, I have taken steps to speak up on behalf of midwives and normal birth. It is not always easy. I wrote comment pieces on breastfeeding and home birth which sparked aggressive online comments from readers (Maclean 2014b, 2014c). It was a weighty responsibility giving a live interview on Sky News, having had no media training, during protests against government plans to axe the NHS bursary for student midwives. Equally, when the *Daily Mail* wanted an interview on the same issue, with photographs of me and my baby son at home, I felt apprehensive. Yet it was a privilege to have exposure to put my case forward. It is often a case of taking small steps. I recently gave Take A Break an interview about a day in my life at work. I described the highs and lows of labour without creating a horror story, and emphasised that a woman's emotional comfort is part of keeping her and the baby safe (Gregory 2017). Getting the piece into print was not without stress, as I had to steer clear of overtly controversial statements out of fairness to my employer. The finished article also made me sound rather cliched. Yet the net result, read by thousands of women, went some way to normalising what it's like to have a baby.

CONCLUSION

Headlines will continue to portray birth as an extreme event, but there is room for fascinating insights into the reality of normal birth too. Midwives are well-placed to provide access to the birthing process, if appropriate media training is given. The RCM has an active press office and this work could be emulated and expanded via NHS maternity departments. If midwives are to fulfil their role as advocates for women under the gaze of an ever-growing media, it is arguably their responsibility to speak up and rewrite the childbirth story.

Editor's Note: Maclean's chapter, looking at representations of labour and childbirth in British newspapers, highlighted that it is not just on television where issues of misrepresentation need to be tackled; newspapers are problematic, too. Maclean argues that midwives need to engage more with media, and notes how her own journalistic experience has helped in some way; but she still cannot get away from the aggressive feedback that engaging the media can provoke, for example, surrounding a topic like breastfeeding. In our next chapter, Catherine Angell, a Senior Academic in Midwifery at Bournemouth University, discusses her research into newspaper representations of infant feeding and the challenges such depictions pose to a woman experiencing both birth and motherhood.

REFERENCES

Adams, S.S., M. Eberhard-Gran, and A. Eskild. 2012. Fear of childbirth and duration of labour: A study of 2206 women with intended vaginal delivery. *BJOG* 119 (10): 1238–1246. doi:10.1111/j.1471-0528.2012.03433.x.

Allan, S. 2010. *News, power and the public sphere, pp. 8–26 of News Culture*. 3rd ed. Maidenhead: McGraw-Hill Education.

Beck, U. 1992. *Risk society: Towards a new modernity*, 46–197. London: Sage.

Bick, D. 2010. Media portrayal of birth and the consequences of misinformation. *Midwifery* 26 (2): 147–148.

Brocklehurst, P., P. Hardy, J. Hollowell, L. Linsell, A. Macfarlane, C. McCourt, et al. 2011. Perinatal and maternal outcomes by planned place of birth for healthy women with low-risk pregnancies: the Birthplace in England national prospective cohort study. *BMJ* 343 (7840): d7400. doi:10.1136/bmj.d7400.

Buse K, Mays N, Walt G. 2012. The health policy framework. Chapter 1 in *Making health policy*, 4–19. London: McGraw-Hill Education.

Cheng, Y.W., J.M. Snowden, S.J. Handler, I.B. Tager, A.E. Hubbard, and A.B. Caughey. 2014. Litigation in obstetrics: Does defensive medicine contribute to increases in cesarean delivery? *The Journal of Maternal-Fetal & Neonatal Medicine* 27 (16): 1668–1675.

Conboy, M. 2011. *Journalism and Political Coverage, pp. 126–130 of Journalism in Britain: A historical introduction*. London: Sage.

Coxon, K, Sandall, J., and Fulop, N. 2014. To what extent are women free to choose where to give birth? How discourses of risk, blame and responsibility influence birth place decisions. *Health, Risk & Society* 16 (1). doi:10.1080/13698575.2013.859231.

Cumberledge, J. 2016. *National Maternity Review. Better Births: Improving outcomes of maternity services in England*. London: The Stationery Office.

Dahlen, H. 2010. Undone by fear? Deluded by trust? *Midwifery* 26 (2): 156–162. doi:10.1016/j.midw.2009.11.008.

Dahlen, H., and C. Homer. 2012. Web-based news reports on midwives compared with obstetricians: A prospective analysis. *Birth* 39 (1): 48–56. doi:10.1111/j.1523-536X.2011.00512.x.

Dick-Read, G. 2004. *Childbirth without fear: The principles and practice of natural childbirth*. London: Pinter & Martin Publishers.

Donnison, J. 1977. *Midwives and medical men: A history of inter-professional rivalries and women's rights.* New York: Schocken.
Dworkin, S., and F. Wachs. 2004. 'Getting your body back'—Postindustrial Fit Motherhood in Shape Fit Pregnancy Magazine. *Gender and Society* 18 (5): 610–624. doi:10.1177/0891243204266817.
Ecker, U.K., S. Lewandowsky, E.P. Chang, and R. Pillai. 2014. The effects of subtle misinformation in news headlines. *Journal of experimental psychology: applied* 20 (4): 323.
Ehrenreich, B., and E. English. 2010. *Witches, midwives, and nurses: A history of women healers*, 2nd ed. New York: Feminist Press.
Farrell, N. 2013. Navigating the stars: The challenges and opportunities of celebrity journalism. In *Journalism: New Challenges*, ed. K. Fowler-Watt, 367–383. Poole: CJCR: Centre for Journalism & Communication Research.
Fenwick, J., J. Gamble, E. Nathan, S. Bayes, and Y. Hauck. 2009. Pre-and postpartum levels of childbirth fear and the relationship to birth outcomes in a cohort of Australian women. *Journal of Clinical Nursing* 18 (5): 667–677. doi:10.1111/j.1365-2702.2008.02568.x.
Fenwick, J., J. Toohill, J. Gamble, D. K. Creedy, A. Buist, E. Turkstra, et al. 2015. Effects of a midwife psycho-education intervention to reduce childbirth fear on women's birth outcomes and postpartum psychological wellbeing. *BMC Pregnancy and Childbirth* 15 (1): 284.
Foucault, M. 1976. *The birth of the clinic*. London: Routledge.
Galtung, J., and M.H. Ruge. 1965. The structure of foreign news: The presentation of the Congo, Cuba and Cyprus crises in four Norwegian newspapers. *Journal of peace research* 2 (1): 64–90.
Gibson, R., and D. Zillmann. 1993. The impact of quotation in news reports on issue perception. *Journalism & Mass Communication Quarterly* 70 (4): 793–800.
Gregory, K. 2017. What it's REALLY like to be an NHS midwife. *Take A Break*. June 22. 26–27.
Haines, H., J.F. Pallant, A. Karlström, and I. Hildingsson. 2011. Crosscultural comparison of levels of childbirth-related fear in an Australian and Swedish sample. *Midwifery* 27 (4): 560–567. doi:10.1016/j.midw.2010.05.004.
Harcup, T., and D. O'neill. 2001. What is news? Galtung and Ruge revisited. *Journalism Studies* 2 (2): 261–280.
Hofberg, K., and M.R. Ward. 2004. Fear of childbirth, tocophobia, and mental health in mothers: The obstetric-psychiatric interface. *Clinical Obstetrics and Gynecology* 47 (3): 527–534.
Hooper, C. 2017. *How to grow a baby and push it out*. London: Vermilion.
Houghton, G., C. Bedwell, M. Forsey, L. Baker, and T. Lavender. 2008. Factors influencing choice in birth place-an exploration of the views of women, their partners and professionals. *Evidence Based Midwifery* 6 (2): 59.

Hundley, V., E. van Teijlingen, and A. Luce. 2015. Do midwives need to be more media savvy? *MIDIRS Midwifery Digest* 25 (1): 5–10.
Janssen, P.A., and S.L. Desmarais. 2013. Women's experience with early labour management at home vs. in hospital: A randomised controlled trial. *Midwifery* 29 (3): 190–194.
Johnson, R., and P. Slade. 2003. Obstetric complications and anxiety during pregnancy: Is there a relationship? *Journal of Psychosomatic Obstetrics and Gynaecology* 24 (1): 1–14.
Jordan, R., and P. Murphy. 2009. Risk assessment and risk distortion: Finding the balance. *J Midwifery Womens Health* 54 (3): 191–200. doi:10.1016/j.jmwh.2009.02.001.
Khan, R., Dawlatly, B., and Chappatte, O. 2013. Pregnancy outcomes following bariatric surgery. *The Obstetrician & Gynaecologist* 15 (1): 37–43.
Kingdon, C. 2009. *The Mass Media in Sociology for Midwives*, 160–186. London: MA Healthcare.
Kitzinger, S. 2012. *The new experience of childbirth*. Hachette, UK.
Knight, M., M. Nair, D. Tuff nell, et al. (eds.). On behalf of MBRRACE-UK. 2016. *Saving lives, improving mothers' care—surveillance of maternal deaths in the UK 2012–14*. Oxford: National Perinatal Epidemiology Unit.
Lacey, N. 2002. *Media institutions and audiences: Key concepts in media studies*. New York: Palgrave.
Larsson, M., G. Aneblom, V. Odlind, and T. Tydén. 2002. Reasons for pregnancy termination, contraceptive habits and contraceptive failure among Swedish women requesting an early pregnancy termination. *Acta Obstetricia et Gynecologica Scandinavica* 81 (1): 64–71.
Leveson, B. 2012. *An inquiry into the culture, practices and ethics of the press: Executive summary and recommendations*, vol. 779. The Stationery Office.
Loewenstein, G., E. Weber, C. Hsee, and N. Welch. 2001. Risk as Feelings. *Psychological Bulletin* 127 (2): 267–286.
Luce, A., M. Cash, V. Hundley, H. Cheyne, E. Van Teijlingen, and C. Angell. 2016. "Is it realistic?" the portrayal of pregnancy and childbirth in the media. *BMC pregnancy and childbirth* 16 (1): 40.
Maclean, E. 2014a. What to expect when you're expecting? Representations of birth in British newspapers. *British Journal of Midwifery* 22 (8).
Maclean, E. 2014b. Breastfeeding versus baby formula is not an either or debate. *Guardian Online*, 3 March 2014. Available at: https://www.theguardian.com/sustainable-business/breastfeeding-formula-debate-mothers-baby. Accessed 23 Aug 2017.
Maclean, E. 2014c. Home birth: Labour in the living room is the sustainable option. *Guardian Online*, 17 May 2014. Available at: https://www.theguardian.com/sustainable-business/home-birth-labour-sustainable-option. Accessed 23 Aug 2017.

McIntyre, M., K. Francis, and Y. Chapman. 2011. Shaping public opinion on the issue of childbirth; a critical analysis of articles published in an Australian newspaper. *BMC Pregnancy Childbirth* 11: 47. doi:10.1186/1471-2393-11-47.

Moorhead, J. 1999. Are you too posh to push? The way you give birth has become a status symbol of our times. And by 2010 half of all women will refuse to endure the pain of natural birth. *Daily Mail*, January 26. 36–37.

National Readership Survey. 2013. *Average Issue Readership—July 2011–June 2012*. London: NRS.

Neilson, J. 2011. *Pre-eclampsia and eclampsia*. Centre for Maternal and Child Enquiries Mission Statement, 66.

NHS. 2016. Hospital Maternity Activity – 2015/16. Available at: http://www.content.digital.nhs.uk/catalogue/PUB22384/hosp-epis-stat-mat-summ-repo-2015-16-rep.pdf. Accessed 13 Feb 2017.

NHS Choices. 2016. Behind the Headlines: Your guide to the science that makes the news. Available online: http://www.nhs.uk/news/Pages/NewsIndex.aspx. Accessed 10 Oct 2016.

NICE. 2014. *CG190 Intrapartum care for healthy women and babies*. London: NICE.

Nolan, M. 2009. Labour isn't happening until health professionals tell you so. In *Early Labour: What's the Problem? Birth*, vol. 36, ed. J. Green, H. Spiby, 332–339.

NPEU. 2010. *Delivered with care: A national survey of women's experience of maternity care*. Oxford: NPEU.

Odent, M. 2013. *Childbirth and the future of Homo sapiens*. Pinter & martin Limited.

RCM. 2012. *Evidence Based Guidelines for Midwifery-Led Care of Women in Labour*. London: RCM.

RCOG. 2015. *SIP 17: The Role of Bariatric Surgery in Improving Reproductive Health*. London: RCOG.

Reah, D. 2002. *The language of newspapers*. Psychology Press.

Renfrew, M. J., A. McFadden, M. H. Bastos, J. Campbell, A. A. Channon, N. F.Cheung, et al. 2014. Midwifery and quality care: findings from a new evidence-informed framework for maternal and newborn care. *The Lancet* 384 (9948): 1129–1145.

Rich, P.R., and M.S. Zaragoza. 2016. The continued influence of implied and explicitly stated misinformation in news reports. *Journal of Experimental Psychology. Learning, Memory, and Cognition* 42 (1): 62.

Robson, S., A. Carey, R. Mishra, and K. Dear. 2008. Elective caesarean delivery at maternal request: A preliminary study of motivations influencing women's decision-making. *Australian and New Zealand Journal of Obstetrics and Gynaecology* 48 (4): 415–420. doi:10.1111/j.1479-828X.2008.00867.x.

Rossignol, M., N. Chaillet, F. Boughrassa, and J.M. Moutquin. 2014. Interrelations between four antepartum obstetric interventions and cesarean delivery in women at low risk: A systematic review and modeling of the cascade of interventions. *Birth* 41 (1): 70–78.

Rouhe, H., K. Salmela-Aro, M. Gissler, E. Halmesmäki, and T. Saisto. 2011. Mental health problems common in women with fear of childbirth. *BJOG* 118 (9): 1104–1111. doi:10.1111/j.1471-0528.2011.02967.x.

Ryding, E., B. Wijma, K. Wijma, and H. Rydhström. 1998. Fear of childbirth during pregnancy may increase the risk of emergency cesarean section. *Acta Obstetricia et Gynecologica Scandinavica* 77 (5): 542–547.

Sandall, J., H. Soltani, S. Gates, A. Shennan, D. Devane. 2016. Midwife-led continuity models versus other models of care for childbearing women. *The Cochrane Library.*

Scamell, M. 2014. Childbirth within the Risk Society. *Sociology Compass* 8 (7): 917–928.

Shennan, A.H., C. Redman, C. Cooper, and F. Milne. 2012. Are most maternal deaths from pre-eclampsia avoidable? *The Lancet* 379 (9827): 1686–1687.

Shennan, A.H., M. Green, and L.C. Chappell. 2017. Maternal deaths in the UK: Pre-eclampsia deaths are avoidable. *The Lancet* 389 (10069): 582–584.

Sundar, S.S. 1998. Effect of source attribution on perception of online news stories. *Journalism & Mass Communication Quarterly* 75 (1): 55–68.

Templeton SK (2012) 'My Baby's Dead, Isn't she Nurse?' A Girl's Death in a Midwife Unit Has Fuelled the Row Over Centres Not Staffed by Obstetricians. 18 November 2012. Available at: http://www.thesundaytimes.co.uk/sto/news/uk_news/Health/article1165213.ece. Accessed 16 Feb 2017.

Tracy, S., and M. Tracy. 2003. Costing the cascade: Estimating the cost of increased obstetrical intervention in childbirth using population data. *BJOG* 110 (8): 717–724.

Tulloch, J., and D. Lupton. 2003. *Risk and everyday life*, 74–123. London: Sage.

Unterscheider, J., M. Ma'Ayeh, and M.P. Geary. 2011. Born before arrival births: Impact of a changing obstetric population. *Journal of Obstetrics and Gynaecology* 31 (8): 721–723.

Young, M., G. Norman, and K. Humphreys. 2008. Medicine in the popular press: The influence of the media on perceptions of disease. *PLoS ONE* 3 (10): e3552. doi:10.1371/journal.pone.0003552.

Zelizer, B. 1989. 'Saying as collective practice: Quoting and differential address in the news. *Text-Interdisciplinary Journal for the Study of Discourse* 9 (5): 369–388.

Zelizer, B, Allan, S. 2010. *Headline—pp. 52–53 in Keywords in news and journalism studies.* Maidenhead: McGraw-Hill Education.

CHAPTER 4

An Everyday Trauma: How the Media Portrays Infant Feeding

Catherine Angell

Abstract Infant feeding is a fundamental element in the childbirth continuum. A woman's decision about whether to breastfeed, and the duration and exclusivity of this, has the potential to affect short and long term health for both herself and her baby (Vitora et al. 2016). When making infant-feeding choices mothers often feel obliged to conform to the expectations of their family, social group and culture (Angell et al. 2011). In addition, women are influenced by the wider society in which they live, and many report feeling pressurized, shamed and marginalised by other people in relation to their infant feeding (Thomson et al. in Maternal & Child Nutrition 11: 33–46, 2015). Although women's choices are essentially personal and private, strong public opinions on the subject transform it into 'everybody's business'. This is exacerbated by mass media, which has become a conduit through which social and individual views on infant feeding are presented and debated. Curiously, the 'everyday' nature of this subject means that it often appears in the media in a covert manner, when it is unconsciously included as a minor element in a wider story. In other cases infant feeding *is* the story, and it

C. Angell (✉)
Bournemouth University, Poole, UK
e-mail: cangell@bournemouth.ac.uk

© The Author(s) 2017
A. Luce et al. (eds.), *Midwifery, Childbirth and the Media*,
DOI 10.1007/978-3-319-63513-2_4

appears in the media as a problematic issue and the focus of discussion (Henderson et al. in British Medical Journal 321: 1196–1198, 2000). During the past two decades a small body of research has emerged which has explored how infant feeding is presented in newspapers, magazines and television, in a range different countries and cultures. This chapter will review the existing literature and consider how the media might influence infant feeding behaviour, both currently and in the future.

Keywords Infant feeding · Motherhood · Newspapers Breastfeeding Media

Infant feeding is an essential aspect of the childbearing cycle and is intrinsically linked to women's experiences of birth and motherhood. Throughout our evolution, and for almost all of human history, breastfeeding has been the mainstay of infant survival (Light 2013). It is, in physiological terms, the normal feeding method for the woman and her baby, and successful breastfeeding enables optimal immediate and long-term health for both (Hoddinott 2008; Horta and Victora 2013). However, the use of formula milks has become very common in high-income countries, and also increasingly in mid- to low-income countries, despite its association with a range of morbidities (Kramer and Kakuma 2007) and infant mortality (Bartick and Reinhold 2010). Although the World Health Organization (WHO) and UNICEF recommend that infants should be exclusively breastfed for at least 6 months, and continue to breastfeed alongside appropriate solid foods to two years of age or beyond (WHO 2003; UNICEF 2013), fewer than 40% of infants worldwide (UNICEF 2013) and under 1% of infants in the UK (McAndrew et al. 2012) experience this.

From a logical perspective, it is perplexing that women and families would make choices that are detrimental to the health of themselves and their children. However, strong forces are at work in influencing women's infant feeding decisions and failure to make substantial impact on these or dramatically improve breastfeeding rates represents a global public health issue (UNICEF 2013). The evidence suggests that this is a multifaceted issue (Sloan 2006); and whilst decisions about whether to start, and when to stop, breastfeeding might be regarded as a personal choice, in reality women must negotiate complex and conflicting pressures. These might include their own personal beliefs about and experience of infant feeding (Andrew and Harvey 2011) and the opinions of their partner, family and friends (Chezem 2003). Women's experience of birth and the effectiveness of the support they receive from professionals and organisations may also have a bearing on feeding choices (Ingram 2013). There is also a recognised impact from product advertising (Parry et al. 2013), social opinions and cultural habits (Scott and Mostyn 2003). All of these outside influences may shape and reinforce women's decisions, but may also aim to censor, shame and marginalise women if their choices do not conform to the expectations of others (Thomson et al. 2015). Of particular interest here are the ways in which the mass media represents infant feeding, and this chapter will draw together the literature looking at media coverage of infant feeding around the world during the last 20 years, illustrated with recent examples from UK media.

It is perhaps surprising that an activity as ordinary and 'everyday' as feeding a baby would elicit any interest at all from those not directly engaged in or affected by it. Yet strong public opinions exist around how babies should be fed, what they should eat and where and when feeding is appropriate (Mannien et al. 2002; Morris et al. 2016). The causes of this public interest are open to speculation, but researchers suggest that contributing factors may include attitudes to female sexuality (Rodriguez-Garcia and Frazier 1995), anxiety around female bodily fluids (Bramwell 2001) and notions of good motherhood (Wall 2001). A brief look at print and broadcast media output reveals an enormous number of infant-feeding-related commentaries and images, suggesting that there is public appetite for the subject. The volume and diversity of this coverage is too great to describe and make sense of in one chapter, but fortunately the phenomenon has been fairly extensively explored in the academic literature, making a literature review a more pragmatic way to explore the subject. Searching the literature reveals over 20 English-language papers, dating from 1999 to 2016, which have investigated representations of infant feeding in printed media (newspapers and magazines) and on television. The media items explored by researchers within these academic papers include news stories, articles, editorials, health columns, adverts, interviews and fictional stories. Researchers have also examined how infant feeding is presented on the Internet (Shaikh and Scott 2005) and in social media (Abrahams 2012), but these are not examined here, because consumers utilise and interact with them in different ways to traditional media (Brossard 2013).

Academic interest in representations of infant feeding in the media emerged nearly two decades ago, when three early publications on the subject emerged in quick succession (Henderson 1999; Henderson et al. 2000; Potter et al. 2000). A steady flow of research has continued since then, so that over 20 papers and theses now exist in the field. These offer considerable variety of approach in terms of location, time span and focus, and provide a rich and informative summary of the history and nature of infant feeding representations in the media. The existing research covers a range (although not a broad range) of locations, such as the United Kingdom (Henderson et al. 2000), the United States (Foss and Southwell 2006), Canada (Potter et al. 2000), Australia (Mannien et al. 2002), Hong Kong (Dodgson et al. 2008) and Malaysia (Mohamad 2011). Whilst most researchers have reported on contemporary media representations there are several who have focused on a longer time frame, with some impressively long periods—examining magazines from 1930 to 2007 (Foss 2010), and from 1945 to 1995 (Potter et al. 2000). The majority of researchers have looked at printed media, whilst some have considered how infant feeding is portrayed in television programmes (Henderson et al. 2000; Brown and Peuchaud 2008; Bridges 2010; Foss 2013). It is worth recognising that, in general, many early researchers in this field tended to undertake broad content analysis of either infant-feeding or breastfeeding coverage in their chosen medium. As time has gone on some have instead focused in on specific aspects of content, such as breastfeeding celebrities (Duvall 2015), human milk sharing (Carter et al. 2015), exclusive breastfeeding (Hamilton and Lewis 2014), environmental risk (Van Esterik 2004) and ethical behaviour in media organisations (Bridges 2007). Focusing on specific topics has enabled a greater level of analysis of the nature of the discourse around infant feeding in the media, increasing our understanding of not only what is being presented but also how it is being presented.

Just this brief resume of the existing literature is sufficient to demonstrate that reviewing every nuance of global media coverage of infant feeding would be an impossible task; indeed, as newspapers, magazines and television churn out their material on a daily basis, and we see ever more stories and commentaries emerging, the task grows ever larger. As such this chapter will focus on the six key themes that underpin much of mass media's coverage of infant feeding.

WHAT'S IN VOGUE?

Researchers exploring long-term patterns in infant-feeding items in the press have concluded that the volume and content of articles and advertisements tend to reflect the fluctuations in the uptake of breastfeeding and formula-milk feeding that have occurred during recent decades. When looking at 50 years of editions of a Canadian women's magazine, Potter et al. (2000) found a move towards pro-breastfeeding items from 1975 onwards, coinciding with the beginning of a swing back to breastfeeding after many years of very high formula-feeding rates. At the same time they also noted a general decrease in infant-feeding content, but this was largely driven by a decline in advertising, which seems to have been a consistent feature in the printed media. Other studies looking at printed media in the United States across long time periods noted similar links between breastfeeding patterns and media content (Foss and Southwell 2006; Foss 2010).

Having noted these temporal trends, it is also if interest to note the findings of research undertaken across a spread of media sources, but on a shorter time scale. Dodgson et al. (2008) identified that both volume and nature of infant-feeding content differed between Chinese- and English-language publications in Hong Kong, with more breastfeeding items found in the English publications, again reflecting social norms and feeding habits within that population. In the United Kingdom researchers have identified that breastfeeding and formula-milk feeding receive a roughly equal amount of coverage, by volume of items, although the balance of these could vary considerably between different publications (Henderson et al. 2000; O'Brien et al. 2016).

The observation that the media tends to be 'in step' with changing breastfeeding and formula-milk-feeding patterns lead us to consider what the mechanism is that links infant-feeding coverage in the media with social trends. An obvious question is whether the media merely follows contemporary public trends and interests in order to appeal to the consumer or proactively drives behaviour change (Seale 2003). Interestingly, in their study of infant-feeding articles between 1972 and 2000, Foss and Southwell (2006) specifically identified media coverage as a driver for behaviour change in infant feeding, arguing that when 'hand feeding' (bottle and solid foods) advertising increased, a decrease in breastfeeding initiation was observed in the following year. Zhang et al. (2013) noted a correlation between women's recollection of seeing formula-milk information in the media and their likelihood of choosing to use formula milk. Contrary to this, one US study found that women believed that the media did not influence their choices (Bylaska-Davies 2015), although the researchers noted that women were aware of various infant-feeding stories in the media. Their view does seem to be at odds with the mainstream of media theory, which broadly agrees, albeit with varying ideas about the actual mechanism, that the media has an influence on public and personal behaviour (Shoemaker and Reese 2013). The nature of this influence, and how it is played out in the media are exemplified by the remaining themes in this chapter.

What's the Message?

In addition to looking at the volume of items relating to breastfeeding or formula-milk feeding portrayed in the media, many researchers have explored the topics covered and the manner in which they were presented. It would seem that few media items, beyond some of those in health columns, are without an element of editorial opinion, which on occasion slips into sensationalism. This is particularly evident in relation to breastfeeding. Identifying underlying influences and motivations in the media can be challenging (Macnamara 2014), but Bridges (2007) comments that media coverage contains "mixed messages and meanings" of which "some are obvious, some are powerful and persuasive, and others subtle but sure" (p. 20). It could be argued that there is an element of 'agenda setting' (McCombs 2013) where the media bring particular issues to the public's attention, thereby creating and perpetuating an issue. This concept has resonance with this issue, as it is perhaps difficult to explain why some infant-feeding media items, particularly news stories, become significant. For example, the UK and US press frequently feature items about women who have been challenged for breastfeeding in public spaces (Angell 2013), or highlight the infant-feeding comments of minor celebrities (O'Brien et al. 2016), resulting in these relatively un-newsworthy events' receiving a disproportionate amount of coverage compared the other news items.

A number of researchers have tried to quantify whether particular infant-feeding media items could be interpreted as positive or negative (Mannien et al. 2002; Dodgson et al. 2008; Bylaska-Davies 2015; O'Brien et al. 2016); and, apart from Bylaska-Davies (2015), all identified that a higher proportion of the media items they reviewed tended to be neutral or positive about breastfeeding than negative. O'Brien et al. (2016) also identified that references to formula-milk feeding were equally positive in nature. However, making judgments about the nature of items was fraught with difficulties. Partly this is because judging whether a story is 'positive' depends on what is being judged. For example, O'Brien et al. (2016) noted a item about a celebrity whose infant would not attach for breastfeeding, which despite appearing rather negative was actually coded as being positive in the way it portrayed 'a combination of feeding methods'. Whether an item is positive or negative also depends on the context of the reader. For example a UK newspaper item describing a woman who was prevented from breastfeeding in a local council office (Narain 2011) includes comments about breastfeeding being 'natural' and 'healthy', which might be construed as positive... but at a different level the story may be seen as negative because it might deter women from breastfeeding if they fear that they too might suffer this kind of embarrassment (Morris et al. 2016). Likewise, celebrity role-modeling of breastfeeding, which may appear to be a potentially positive influence in encouraging other women to breastfeed, may in fact backfire if other women perceive that only the affluent are likely to breastfeed (O'Brien et al. 2016). The inevitable conclusion drawn by researchers in this field is that media coverage of infant feeding is characterized by mixed messages and ambiguous intentions.

STEREOTYPING

Infant-feeding items in the media illustrate a range of social, cultural and racial stereotypes. It has long been recognised that in high income countries women who are more affluent and educated have a greater propensity to initiate breastfeeding than other women (Kelly and Watt 2005). In the media breastfeeding items frequently only relate to 'middle-class', well-off women (Henderson et al. 2000) or celebrities (Duvall 2015). By contrast, formula-milk feeding is portrayed as something that 'ordinary' families do (Henderson et al. 2000). In fictional television breastfeeding can be identified as a signifier of social class (Henderson et al. 2000), and where women do not exemplify the assumed breastfeeding demographic, this is noted and commented on (Foss 2013). Foss (2013) also noted a preponderance of white women engaged in breastfeeding in US television programmes, compared to women of other ethnicities. What is perhaps more sinister are instances noted by researchers where there is an asymmetrical coverage of infant feeding amongst women of different social and ethnic groups, with sympathy for women in the 'standard' breastfeeding demographic who experience feeding problems, and harsh criticism for those who, because of their social or racial group, do not 'fit' social expectations (Brown and Peuchaud 2008).

Ordinary or Extraordinary?

Whilst breastfeeding is the normal way to feed an infant it is generally acknowledged that a considerable number of women and babies experience common breastfeeding problems, such as sore nipples, engorgement, mastitis and concern about milk volume (Bergmann et al. 2014); and women may also have a baby who struggles to feed effectively due to prematurity, jaundice or tongue-tie (Wambach and Riordan 2014). Whilst infant-feeding problems are the subject of real-life and fictional media items, several researchers note that these constituted a fairly small proportion of items (Dodgson et al. 2008; Foss 2013; O'Brien et al. 2016), potentially leading to false expectations about the breastfeeding experience (Foss 2010). Within the limited discussion of feeding problems in the media the number of breastfeeding difficulties outnumbered those relating to issues with formula-milk feeding (Henderson et al. 2000). This largely reflects the reality of feeding, but when it is presented without discussion around the health risks of formula feeding, it may be difficult for audiences to put media items about breastfeeding difficulties into context. The experience of normal breastfeeding problems portrayed on television is identified as being associated with high emotion, weeping and pain (Foss 2013). Where problems were presented there was rarely factual information about resolving them, beyond the need for time and practice (Henderson et al. 2000; Foss 2010, 2013; O'Brien et al. 2016). The overall message mothers receive may be that breastfeeding is a difficult and problematic activity, at which they may fail (Henderson et al. 2000; Potter et al. 2000; Frerichs et al. 2006), as well as being inconvenient and restrictive (Foss 2013).

However, perhaps the most concerning aspect of media coverage, in terms of presenting breastfeeding as a normal behaviour, is the focus on two extreme aspects of feeding—lactation related comedy and infant death. Henderson (2000) identified the tendency of British television to present breastfeeding as funny or embarrassing, with portrayals of the 'out of control' female body. Even the title of Foss's paper 'That's not a Beer Bong, It's a Breast Pump' (Foss 2013) encapsulates the common theme of breastfeeding being absurd or humorous in the media. It could be argued that society finds humour here because breastfeeding women do not conform to the accepted ideals of the normal or attractive female body, perhaps fitting the category of women described by Rowe (2007) as 'associated with dirt, liminality (thresholds, borders or margins) and taboo, rendering above all a figure of ambivalence' (Rowe 2007, p. 261).

Alarmingly, because extreme events are newsworthy, and provide compelling storylines, there is also a tendency for the media to pick up on the rare but tragic results of breastfeeding problems. Several researchers noted examples in the media of real and fictional examples of infants dying as a result of ineffective, deviant or negligent breastfeeding (Henderson et al. 2000; Brown and Peuchaud 2008; Foss 2013) or being harmed by women's use of illegal substances (Foss 2013) or pollutants (Van Esterik 2004). Hausman comments that 'to a public whose model is formula feeding, it can seem as if ordinary breastfeeding itself results in dead babies' (Hausman 2003, p. 37).

A HEALTHY CHOICE

The identification of tragedy related to infant feeding leads naturally into exploring how the media portray the health risks and benefits of breastfeeding and formula milk. The commonly used term 'benefits of breastfeeding' suggests that breastfeeding is a 'value added' choice. This is a modern concept, because until the twentieth century breastfeeding (either by mother or wet nurse) was regarded as the only safe means to feed a baby rather than being merely 'beneficial'. To try to return to this idea of breastfeeding as the physiological norm, health professionals have recently tried to move the discourse to focus on the risks of formula milk feeding rather than the benefits of breastfeeding (McNiel et al. 2010). However, much of the literature in this review still discusses the issue from the 'breastfeeding benefits' angle. Several existing research papers have identified the lack of information about the benefits of breastfeeding (Henderson et al. 2000; Frerichs et al. 2006; Foss 2013), although items presenting breastfeeding as effective for weight loss (O'Brien et al. 2016) and 'best for baby' (Foss 2010) were identified by some researchers. In their Hong Kong study, Dodgson et al. (2008) note that value of breast milk, in terms of nutrition and/or other health benefits for the baby, were identified in around a quarter of media items. Foss (2013) suggests that the presence of breastfeeding stereotypes may be a barrier to elucidating the benefits of breastfeeding, because no explanations of feeding choice are required for such women, beyond fitting into a recognised social group.

It has already been noted that formula-milk feeding is frequently mentioned in contemporary media items, despite its known associations with suboptimal health. Hence it is perhaps remarkable that some researchers have identified that perceived benefits of formula milk, particularly the potential for fathers to feed the baby (O'Brien et al. 2016), may be presented more frequently than the risks (Dodgson et al. 2008), which may be limited to practical issues such as the time required to make up feeds (Henderson et al. 2000). In addition, the risks of formula feeding may be highlighted less often than the potential risks of breastfeeding (Henderson et al. 2000). Indeed, on occasion, the rare or risks of breastfeeding, such as environmental contaminants (Van Esterik 2004) or insufficient milk (Henderson et al. 2000; Brown and Peuchaud 2008; Foss 2013) presented in the media may skew the debate to the extent that formula feeding appears to be a healthier choice. Most researchers note that the media could be a hugely powerful instrument with which to promote effective breastfeeding (Henderson 1999; Henderson et al. 2000; Mannien et al. 2002; Foss 2013; O'Brien et al. 2016) but media organisations, as Brown and Peuchaud (2008) comment 'are not in the business of health education'.

Breastfeeding in the Public Gaze

The final theme in the literature focuses on breastfeeding in public spaces, which is a recurring subject in the media (Mannien et al. 2002). It would be difficult to overstate media interest in this activity, which has been identified as a common and recurring theme that brings together many of society's insecurities around bodily fluids, sexuality and female roles. It is perhaps here that the concept of 'mixed messages' in the media is most apparent. In essence news reports about women being harassed when breastfeeding suggest that the media aims to highlight their plight. However, whilst this has raised the question of protection for breastfeeding in public spaces in the United Kingdom, Australia and the US (Boyer 2012) it also presents breastfeeding as a limiting and potentially embarrassing activity (Angell 2013). In addition, these news items stimulate public debate about the issue that demonstrates attitudes which are intolerant and can often be broadly critical of breastfeeding mothers, both in relation to feeding in public spaces and in terms of their general behaviour (Hamilton and Lewis 2014). This dichotomy extends to celebrity mothers, whose breastfeeding choice may lead them to be praised as good mothers, but criticized for being seen undertaking activities which are perceived as intimate or even "offensive" (Bridges 2007) or, in the case of breastfeeding another woman's child or a toddler, undertaking an activity that is "deviant" (Duvall 2015). Fictional stories in the media also frequently pick up the theme of breastfeeding in public spaces, and Foss (2013) presents a number of examples of scenes in which women were either heavily criticized or subjected to prejudice or sexual innuendo. Henderson et al. (2000) identified that in their UK study breastfeeding was referred to in 10 fictional scenes on television, compared to formula-milk feeding, which was included in 170 scenes. Furthermore, whilst formula milk was usually visually present as a background aspect to the scene, breastfeeding was "usually subject to remark" (Henderson et al. 2000).

The flip side of the debate around breastfeeding in public spaces, which is so actively played out in the media, is the paucity of images actually depicting breastfeeding (O'Brien et al. 2016). Indeed, in the United States there were no visual depictions of breastfeeding on US television until 1994 (Foss 2013). Mannien et al. (2002) noted that in their review of the Australian press only 1.3% of articles included a photograph of a breastfeeding baby and a study of British women's magazines pointed out that of 12 infant-feeding images, only one depicted breastfeeding (O'Brien et al. 2016). This perhaps reflects Western society's discomfort with images of 'the breastfeeding breast' (Bridges 2007) compared to the more common imagery of the 'sexual breast' (Duvall 2015). This perpetuates breastfeeding as a hidden practice (Henderson et al. 2000), further inhibiting breastfeeding in public spaces, rather than enabling it to become 'normal and ordinary' (Bylaska-Davies 2015).

Conclusions

This chapter has reviewed the history and current status of infant feeding in the mass media, with reference to the body of work created by researchers and commentators in this field. It is clear that the conclusion drawn in one of the earliest papers—that the media's coverage amounts to "mixed messages" (Henderson 1999), still has resonance, despite having been published almost 20 years ago. A growing acceptance of the evidence that breastfeeding is a healthy behaviour struggles against deep-seated social ambivalence. When combined with the media's desire to provide entertainment through drama, scandal and tragedy, this creates a confusing discourse. In doing so it fails to portray the facts around infant feeding accurately, simultaneously under-representing the risks of formula-milk feeding and discouraging the acceptance of breastfeeding as a normal, 'everyday' activity.

Editor's Note: Angell has explored the complicated discourses around breastfeeding and its representation in British newspapers in this chapter. She highlights the confusion that occurs when the media provides entertainment through drama and tragedy. Alexia Leachman, creator of the Fear Free Childbirth podcast understands this all too well. In our next chapter, Leachman explores her path to motherhood and how she conquered her own fears around childbirth and early labour and how she has gone on to help and support thousands of women through their own pregnancy journeys.

REFERENCES

Abrahams, S.W. 2012. Milk and social media online communities and the International Code of Marketing of Breast-milk Substitutes. *Journal of Human Lactation* 28 (3): 400–406.
Andrew, N., and K. Harvey. 2011. Infant feeding choices: Experience, self-identity and lifestyle. *Maternal & Child Nutrition* 7 (1): 48–60.
Angell, C. 2013. Bare necessities: Why does society make breastfeeding so complicated? *The Practising Midwife* 16 (3): 5.
Bartick, M., and A. Reinhold. 2010. The burden of suboptimal breastfeeding in the United States: A pediatric cost analysis. *Pediatrics* 125 (5): e1048–e1056.
Bergmann, R.L., K.E. Bergmann, K. von Weizsacker, M. Berns, W. Henrich, and J.W. Dudenhausen. 2014. Breastfeeding is natural but not always easy: Intervention for common medical problems of breastfeeding mothers—A review of the scientific evidence. *Journal of Perinatal Medicine* 42 (1): 9–18.
Boyer, K. 2012. Affect, corporeality and the limits of belonging: Breastfeeding in public in the contemporary UK. *Health & Place* 18 (3): 552–560.
Bramwell, R. 2001. Blood and milk: Constructions of female bodily fluids in Western society. *Women and Health* 34 (4): 85–96.
Bridges, N. 2007. Ethical responsibilities of the Australian media in the representations of infant feeding. *Breastfeeding Review* 15 (1): 17.
Bridges, N. 2010. Breastfeeding in the Australian media. *Public Communication Review* 1 (1): 57–64.

Brossard, D. 2013. New media landscapes and the science information consumer. *Proceedings of the National Academy of Sciences* 110 (Supplement 3): 14096–14101.
Brown, J.D., and S.R. Peuchaud. 2008. Media and breastfeeding: Friend or foe? *International Breastfeeding Journal* 3 (1): 1–3.
Bylaska-Davies, P. 2015. Exploring the effect of mass media on perceptions of infant feeding. *Health Care for Women International* 36 (9): 1056–1070.
Carter, S.K., B. Reyes-Foster, and T.L. Rogers. 2015. Liquid gold or Russian roulette? Risk and human milk sharing in the US news media. *Health, Risk & Society* 17 (1): 30–45.
Chezem, J., C. Friesen, and J. Boettcher. 2003. Breastfeeding knowledge, breastfeeding confidence, and infant feeding plans: Effects on actual feeding practices. *Journal of Obstetric, Gynecologic, and Neonatal Nursing* 32 (1): 40–47.
Dodgson, J.E., M. Tarrant, J.T. Thompson, and B. Young. 2008. An analysis of infant feeding content found within the Hong Kong print media. *Journal of Human Lactation* 24 (3): 317–325.
Duvall, S.-S. 2015. Not "Simply the Breast" Media discourses of celebrity, breastfeeding, and normalcy. *Feminist Media Studies* 15 (2): 324–340.
Foss, K.A. 2010. Perpetuating "scientific motherhood": Infant feeding discourse in Parents magazine, 1930–2007. *Women and Health* 50 (3): 297–311.
Foss, K.A. 2013. "That's not a beer bong, it's a breast pump!" Representations of breastfeeding in prime-time fictional television. *Health Communication* 28 (4): 329–340.
Foss, K.A., and B.G. Southwell. 2006. Infant feeding and the media: The relationship between Parents' Magazine content and breastfeeding, 1972–2000. *International Breastfeedinf Journal* 1.
Frerichs, L., J.L. Andsager, S. Campo, M. Aquilino, and C.S. Dyer. 2006. Framing breastfeeding and formula-feeding messages in popular U.S. magazines. *Women and Health* 44 (1): 95–118.
Hamilton, A.E., and M. Lewis. 2014. Exclusive breastfeeding and breastfeeding in newspapers: Analysis of frames, content, and valence. *Proceedings of the New York State Communication Association* 2013 (2013): 5.
Hausman, B.L. 2003. *Mother's milk: Breastfeeding controversies in American culture*. Hove: Psychology Press.
Henderson, A. 1999. Mixed messages about the meaning of breast-feeding representations in the Australian press and popular magazines. *Midwifery* 15 (1): 24–31.
Henderson, L., J. Kitzinger, and J. Green. 2000. Representing infant feeding: Content analysis of British media portrayal of bottle-feeding and breastfeeding. *British Medical Journal* 321: 1196–1198.
Hoddinott, P., D. Tappin, and C. Wright. 2008. Breastfeeding. *British Medical Journal* 336: 881–887.

Horta, B.L., and C.G. Victora. 2013. Long-term effects of breastfeeding—A systematic review.
Ingram, J. 2013. A mixed methods evaluation of peer support in Bristol, UK: Mothers', midwives' and peer supporters' views and the effects on breastfeeding. *BMC Pregnancy and Childbirth, 13*.
Kelly, Y., and R. Watt. 2005. Breast-feeding initiation and exclusive duration at 6 months by social class: results from the Millennium Cohort Study. *Public Health Nutrition* 8 (4): 417–421.
Kramer, M.S. and R. Kakuma. 2007. Optimal duration of exclusive breastfeeding. *Cochrane Database of Systematic Reviews* (4), CD003517.
Light, E.C. 2013. Ancient bodies, modern lives: How evolution has shaped women's health. *Neonatal Network* 32 (2): 138.
Macnamara, J. 2014. *Journalism and PR: Unpacking 'spin'*. Stereotypes and Media Myths: Peter Lang.
Mannien, J., W.E. van den Brandhof, J.E. Hiller, and E. McIntyre. 2002. Breastfeeding articles in the Australian press: 1996–1999. *Breastfeeding Review* 10 (1): 5.
McAndrew, F., J. Thompson, L. Fellows, A. Large, M. Speed, and M.J. Renfrew. 2012. *Infant feeding survey 2010*. Leeds: Health and Social Care Information Centre.
McCombs, M. 2013. *Setting the agenda: The mass media and public opinion*. London: Wiley.
McNiel, M.E., M.H. Labbok, and S.W. Abrahams. 2010. What are the risks associated with formula feeding? A re-analysis and review. *Birth* 37 (1): 50–58.
Mohamad, E. 2011. *Breastfeeding, media and culture: Negotiating space, modesty, motherhood and risk in Malaysia*. Cardiff: Cardiff University.
Morris, C., G.A.Z. de la Fuente, C.E. Williams, and C. Hirst. 2016. UK views toward breastfeeding in public an analysis of the public's response to the Claridge's incident. *Journal of Human Lactation*, http://dx.doi.org/10.1177/0890334416648934.
Narain, J. 2011. *Breastfeeding mother 'told to leave council headquarters because it is a multicultural building'*, vol. 13 July. London: Daily Mail.
O'Brien, E., P. Myles, and C. Pritchard. 2016. The portrayal of infant feeding in British women's magazines: A qualitative and quantitative content analysis. *Journal of Public Health*, https://doi.org/10.1093/pubmed/fdw024.
Parry, K., E. Taylor, P. Hall-Dardess, M. Walker, and M. Labbok. 2013. Understanding women's interpretations of infant formula advertising. *Birth* 40 (2): 115–124.
Potter, B., J. Sheeshka, and R. Valaitis. 2000. Content analysis of infant feeding messages in a Canadian women's magazine, 1945 to 1995. *Journal of Nutrition Education* 32, 196–203.

Rodriguez-Garcia, R., and L. Frazier. 1995. Cultural paradoxes relating to sexuality and breastfeeding. *Journal of Human Lactation* 11 (2): 111–115.
Rowe, K. 2007. *The unruly woman. Understanding inequality: The intersection of race/ethnicity, class, and gender*, 261. Lanham: Rowman & Littlefield.
Scott, J., and T. Mostyn. 2003. Women's experiences of breastfeeding in a bottle–Feeding culture. *Journal of Human Lactation* 19 (3): 270–277.
Seale, C. 2003. Health and media: An overview. *Sociology of Health & Illness* 25 (6): 513–531.
Shaikh, U., and B.J. Scott. 2005. Extent, accuracy, and credibility of breastfeeding information on the Internet. *Journal of Human Lactation* 21 (2): 175–183.
Shoemaker, P. J., and S.D. Reese. 2013. *Mediating the message in the 21st century: A media sociology perspective*. Abingdon: Routledge.
Sloan, S., H. Sneddon, M. Stewart, and D. Iwaniec. 2006. Breast is best? Reasons why mothers decide to breastfeed or bottlefeed their babies and factors influencing the duration of breastfeeding. *Journal of Child Care in Practice* 12 (3): 283–297.
Thomson, G., K. Ebisch-Burton, and R. Flacking. 2015. Shame if you do– Shame if you don't: Women's experiences of infant feeding. *Maternal & child nutrition* 11 (1): 33–46.
UNICEF. 2013. *Breastfeeding on the worldwide agenda*. Available from https://www.unicef.org/eapro/breastfeeding_on_worldwide_agenda.pdf. Accessed March 2017.
Van Esterik, P. 2004. Are media putting infants at risk? Environmental risks, breast feeding and the media. *Women and Environments International* 42: 43.
Wall, G. 2001. Moral constructions of motherhood in breastfeeding discourse. *Gender & Society* 15 (4): 592–610.
Wambach, K., and J. Riordan. 2014. *Breastfeeding and human lactation*. Burlington: Jones & Bartlett Publishers.
WHO. 2003. *Global strategy for infant and young child feeding*. London: World Health Organisation.
Zhang, Y., E. Carlton, and S.B. Fein. 2013. The association of prenatal media marketing exposure recall with breastfeeding intentions, initiation, and duration. *Journal of Human Lactation*, http://dx.doi.org/10.1177/0890334413487256.

CHAPTER 5

How Media Promote Fear Around Childbirth

Alexia Leachman

Abstract Leachman discusses how new media have an opportunity to interrupt the fear-mongering pattern of traditional media to change how women feel about birth. Leachman uses her experience of her Fear Free Childbirth podcast to explain how new media represents an opportunity for women's perceptions of birth to be challenged in a positive way. Her podcast, which has been downloaded over 300,000 times worldwide, helps women around the world to unlearn their childbirth fears and helps them to prepare for a positive birth experience. The podcast does this through sharing extensive interviews with birth professionals and experts, positive birth stories told by the mothers themselves and Leachman helping mothers to shift their mindset around birth. Leachman argues that media need to take responsibility for their reluctant role in educating women on pregnancy and childbirth. Leachman discusses how the portrayal of birth in the media currently tends toward the negative or frivolous, and how information that can help women to prepare in a meaningful way is widely lacking. Through her work as a therapeutic coach, she witnesses first hand how the childbirth myths

---

A. Leachman (✉)
Gothic House, Barker Gate, Nottingham, UK
e-mail: alexia@fearfreechildbirth.com

© The Author(s) 2017
A. Luce et al. (eds.), *Midwifery, Childbirth and the Media*,
DOI 10.1007/978-3-319-63513-2_5

perpetuated by the media are feeding women's fears around birth. She explores some common childbirth fears and some of these fears can lead to traumatic birth experiences, and the potential consequences for family health and wellbeing. Given the impact that fear has on birth, Leachman calls for more to be done to educate women. She explains that this can be done creatively in ways that will engage and have impact, and that the media are well-placed to have a part to play in a broader integrated solution in helping women to birth without fear.

Keywords Podcast · Fear · Childbirth · Pain-free birth · Myths

INTRODUCTION

The day I found out I was pregnant for the first time was a very dark day. I was in shock. The pregnancy wasn't planned, but it wasn't that—I was terrified at the thought of giving birth. I didn't have any friends with children so my knowledge about childbirth was limited to what I'd learnt at school and what I had picked up through life. What I didn't realize was that I had tokophobia, an extreme fear of pregnancy and birth.

In my first trimester, to help me cope with the idea of giving birth, I decided I would opt for an elective C-section. I simply could not contemplate the thought of going through the painful experience that was waiting for me. At the end of my first trimester, I was told it was possible to experience a pain-free birth without pain medication. At first I thought they were pulling my leg—this was news to me. This prompted a burst of childbirth education on my part as I sought to understand how pain-free birth could be possible.

Whilst researching, I learnt how fear increases the experience of pain during childbirth and this led to an epiphany: *if I could clear my fears, then maybe I could have a pain-free birth*. I had just trained in a newly launched therapy and I decided that I would use this therapy to clear my fears. I spent my second trimester clearing my fears and in my seventh month, I changed my birth plan to a home birth. My birth was everything that I had worked hard towards: relatively short at under six hours and pain-free.

After I managed to repeat my positive, pain-free birth experience for the second time, I was approached by friends of friends. They had heard about my journey, overcoming my fears to have a positive birth, and they wanted to know how I'd done it. The quantity of emails I was receiving soon got to the point that I decided it would be quicker to write a book, which I did while nursing my newborn. However, I wanted to get this information out quicker than publishing a book would enable me to do, so I launched my Fear Free Childbirth podcast as a little maternity project.

My aim with the podcast was to share information and inspiration about pregnancy and birth that would help to alleviate the fear that so many women feel about birth. I wanted to provide the information that I wished I could have had access to. I had every intention of doing just one season and going back to my business at the time. But that was not to be.

The success of the podcast caught me off guard, and what started as a need to share important information quickly became my work as I was soon inundated with emails from women around the world letting me know how my podcast was helping them to shift their mindset around birth and have positive birth experiences. My inbox is full of emails like this:

… your podcasts and website have changed my life. I found out I was pregnant, 1 week before my 31st birthday and even though I am in a stable relationship and was planning children in the future, it was a total shock and I went into meltdown mode. I was eventually diagnosed with pre-natal depression and I was hating being pregnant and I felt very alone. I took time off work, went into my shell and my poor fiancée didn't know what do to support me. I was scared of everything to do with the baby, pregnancy, childbirth, my guilt for not feeling happy like a 'normal' pregnant woman should and it was a horrible time. Then I discovered your podcast. That was week 16 of my pregnancy and since then (I am now 23 weeks) I have not been able to get enough of your content. I listen to your podcasts (again and again) on the bus. It has changed my outlook on everything and I am starting to feel in control of my body and mind again.

Thank you for all your work and the positive influence you have had on me. You have enabled my empowerment as a pregnant woman! Thank you, thank you, thank you!! Xxx

I wanted to send you a message to tell you how much your podcast helped me to have a wonderful experience of pregnancy and childbirth. I was anxious to pursue a fear-free, minimal intervention birth, but also overwhelmed with negative advice and opinions. Your podcast was so positive and inspiring and it helped me find the mindset and confidence I needed to have the experience for which I had hoped. My labor was honestly a magical experience. It felt to me like some huge and divine force moved into my body and made the process happen ... I was able to avoid all medical interventions. I was in my "oxytocin bubble," as I called it, with my loving husband, reassuring doula, calming nurse, and kick-ass midwife. I caught my own daughter in the birthing tub and brought her to the surface and into my arms. I know a lot of my positive attitude and, as my midwife called it, "stick-to-it-iveness, to this podcast! Thank you! Please keep doing this wonderful work! I tell every woman I know about this podcast."

At the time of writing, the podcast is in its third season and combines three strands: (1) real-life positive birth stories told by real women; (2) interviews with birth professionals and experts, and (3) advice and strategies on reducing fear and boosting a positive birth mindset. Since its launch, the podcast has been downloaded over 300,000 times and is listened to in over 175 countries.

The presence of fear among pregnant women was far more common than I anticipated, which led me to change the focus of my therapy and coaching work. Now I focus entirely on supporting women on their pregnancy and birth journey. Since I began working with pregnant women, I've discovered that my experience as a fearful pregnant woman was not as unusual as I originally thought. My assumptions around birth are very widespread among women, at least among those that get in touch with me. So why is this?

The elephant in the room here is this: how could I, a university-educated, 36-year-old professional, get to this point in life and NOT know some of these basic facts about birth?

My first memory of learning about childbirth age 13 was a video of a birth in a biology class. It was a hospital scene of a woman lying on her back, screaming. There were staff in white coats and there was a lot of blood. I don't recall learning much else about birth at the time, but I'm very clear on the impact of that video; it was the only contraception I needed because I didn't want to go through that. This video haunted me and steered me successfully away from having kids.

For as long as I can remember, I believed that birth happened in a hospital and that it was a dramatic, scary and painful event in a woman's life. My childbirth education did not include any other variations of birth, so I had no idea that birth could be calm, pleasurable or euphoric, or that it could happen just as easily at home. As my life progressed, my views of childbirth were never challenged; if anything they were reinforced by images and stories of childbirth portraying this dramatic, painful and scary event. Whether it was through film storylines, or headline-grabbing personal stories in magazines and newspapers, the consistent theme was the same: childbirth is painful. Was it any surprise that I was scared? I had every right to be. But that wasn't the only reason I was scared. Being pregnant forced me to examine more closely what my issues with childbirth and my fears were. Clearly I had absorbed this idea of childbirth subconsciously, not through a deliberate or proactive attempt to learn about birth, but from mainstream societal and cultural messages. So what were those messages?

What Society Teaches Women About Birth

If a girl grows up without any positive role model when it comes to birth education, then she will build up a picture about birth from her culture. In the Western world, the media is at the centre of that world. The overarching message that the media teaches us about birth is that it's painful, but that's not all. In a relentless fashion, women are exposed to many other myths about birth that are very narrow in focus while also being incredibly damaging. Here are some of the common childbirth myths that we are being fed both explicitly and subtly.

Childbirth Will Be Painful

This is always presented as an undeniable fact. It just hurts. Even worse, the word "childbirth" is often used interchangeably with the word "pain", and we're never too far from a goading headline that report experiences that are more painful than childbirth. It's the gold standard when it comes to pain.

Birth Is a Medical Process that Needs to Happen in a Hospital

This is very far from what birth actually is—a natural process that leads to better outcomes in a private, homely setting. Sadly, some women don't even realise that birth can happen at home. When I shared with colleagues that I was planning a home birth, I was repeatedly asked, "Why? Isn't there a hospital where you live?" This question exposes this myth beautifully.

Women Give Birth on Their Backs

King Louis XIV of France has been famously attributed to starting this trend because he wanted to watch his mistress give birth to their son. Remarkably, this practice continues to this day, despite the lack of evidence that it is beneficial. Quite the opposite, when women are on their back it increases the need for the very interventions that the doctors claim to want to avoid. The fact that this practice continues today raises many questions, but the real problem is that it forms part of the widespread belief that giving birth is painful because of the way birth is portrayed in the media with the woman on her back. As a result, most people merely accept this as how things supposed to be done. Many women's fears can be attributed to this alone, so the psychological impact of this myth must not be underestimated.

One very common fear that I help women with concerns loss of control. As their pregnancy progresses, they "lose" control of their body as the natural process marches on to its inevitable conclusion. Add to this is the inescapability of the experience, and women can very easily feel trapped, which is another thing I hear a lot. Once pregnant, there is no real escape: you're in it for the long haul until the birth. This combination of loss of control and feeling trapped can have a quite powerful and negative impact on pregnant women.

Lying on your back is a vulnerable position for anyone, with most people only feeling safe enough to do so in the privacy and safety of their own homes. If we have women who are already struggling with feelings around loss of control or feelings of being trapped, then being encouraged, perhaps against their will, to be on their back may exacerbate these fears. Add to this the physical and emotional demands of labour, perhaps for extended periods, and it's not hard to understand why this practice might be psychologically challenging for women.

Strangers Will Look at Your Privates

Whenever a birth is portrayed on TV or in films, there is always an audience. We very rarely just see the woman on her own with her husband. If we consider that the woman might already be feeling vulnerable due to being in labour and being encouraged to be on her back, and you add a loss of respect with an audience of strangers looking at your privates into the mix, it's clear how the resulting emotional stress would not be conducive to positive birth outcomes.

Women Need Help to Give Birth; They Can't Do It on Their Own

Whether they are led to believe that they need the help of an army of medical staff, or they need assistance in the form of medication or machines, the message is the same: women are not capable of doing this on their own. Until the late nineteenth century women gave birth for thousands of years very successfully "on their own"; we wouldn't all be here otherwise! The support that counts is the emotional support that has been provided by women in the community since the beginning of time. But today, the message is clear: women need help to give birth.

Other People "Deliver" the Baby

Whenever we read about births happening in random, unexpected places such as the side of the road, on a plane or in a lift, the headline will usually refer to the passerby who stepped in and "delivered" the baby. No credit is given to the mother who birthed her baby.

The underlying message here is that birth *happens to* a woman, she doesn't take an active, central role and is not the person "doing" it. This sets a woman up to give her power to other people during her pregnancy and birth—this can have a lasting negative impact on her birth experience. By seeing birth as something that "happens" to her she perhaps might not choose to take an active role in her birth education and in doing so expose herself to the possibility of a negative birth experience.

I have detailed all these myths as a result of a very conscious and deliberate process of helping myself try to figure out why I was so fearful. Many women will not go through this questioning and exploratory process, but will simply try to navigate their pregnancy as best they can assuming that what they've been lead to believe about birth is true.

During both of my pregnancies I was hungry for useful information, but this was hard to come by. Most information available is superficial and distracting and doesn't help a pregnant woman become well informed or empowered—quite the opposite. Pregnant women are faced with a very depressing choice when it comes to information about pregnancy and birth as, predictably, they are being fed the usual fodder: fear based, consumer oriented or focused on enhancing one's appearance. Typical headlines include—

- Foods to avoid during pregnancy.
- Top pregnancy exercises to help you bounce back more easily after birth.
- How to look hot in maternity clothes.
- Beauty must-buys for glowing pregnancy skin.
- My birth horror story.
- This season's must-have pram.
- Pinterest boards for beautiful nurseries.

Unfortunately, very little of this is helpful to a woman who wants to prepare for a positive birth experience. She needs to learn about things that can really make a difference to her birth experience: birth choices available to her, how to manage labour pain, the risks and benefits of various medical interventions and how she can best prepare for birth itself. Unfortunately, it is easy to find scare-mongering information or trivial tidbits of information, but difficult to obtain intelligent, well-thought-through or balanced information that would enable a woman to make the choice that was right for her. The only way I was able to make informed decisions during my pregnancy was to read copious amounts of research and policy papers. These are not written with the pregnant mother in mind, and so this was not an easy task.

A lot of what I learnt made it onto the podcast. I remember being desperately angry that important information wasn't easily available. Information that I felt I should have had access to. When you're pregnant you're faced with many choices and some difficult decisions. These decisions might be life changing, and you have to live with the consequences for the rest of your life. And yet, help in evaluating your options and understanding the benefits and risks of various choices is distinctly lacking.

One common theme that emerged from my work with women is the volume of fear-based messages they feel bombarded with when it comes to pregnancy and birth. I frequently receive emails from listeners thanking me for helping them to unlearn what they've learnt elsewhere, with many stating how my podcast is helping to repair the damage that TV shows like *One Born Every Minute* has had on them.

One Born Every Minute is probably one of the most widely known TV shows about birth. It is a reality show that has been edited to maximize the drama in a way which I believe is responsible for creating a lot of fear in women. Many of the birth professionals I speak to recommend that pregnant women do not watch it while pregnant. I believe that women choose to watch it because of the lack of better TV shows about birth. They watch it in the belief that it is a fair representation of birth and that it's helping them to prepare. Little do they realise that by watching repeated versions of dramatic, highly medicalised births, they're stimulating the reticular-activating system in their brain. This is like our internal satellite navigation that brings us closer to the goals we set ourselves. We can consciously choose the goal and then support our choice through education, visualization and action. I hear many women say that their birth plan was to "go with the flow" or "to wing it". This is a clear case of not consciously choosing a goal. In this instance, the brain will assume that what you want is the thing you focus your attention on; and if this is fear-based and/or dramatic or medicalised birth, then this is more likely to be the outcome.

If a woman wants to truly learn about birth then she must pay for her education, whether it be for (a) private antenatal classes, (b) books or (c) paid-for documentaries such as *The Business of Being Born, Beautiful Births Documentary* or *Microbirth*. Childbirth education is distinctly lacking in the Western world, and unfortunately mainstream media is filling the gap. In an ideal world boys and girls would receive a solid education around pregnancy and birth at school as this would not only help to prepare the pregnant women of tomorrow, but also help dads-to-be to feel better informed and thus prepared—they feel fear too!

Media as Birth Educators

The problem with mainstream media stepping in as childbirth educators is the conflict in objectives. Childbirth education aims to help women understand birth and the choices they face; the media is chasing subscribers or advertising money. Media is less concerned with whether what it presents is factual, evidence-based or helpful than with ratings and advertising money: this gives rise to headline-grabbing themes which necessitates drama and fear-based messages. Fear-based messages have no place in effective childbirth education due to the negative role that fear has on birth. I invited Professor Hannah Dahlen (see also Chap. 8) onto my podcast to discuss her research into childbirth education. She believes that "fear is the enemy of birth" because "a woman who is scared will not labour well". Dahlen also stated that "fear is culturally constructed" and that "media reflects and creates our reality".

Research tells us that when fear is present during labour, birth is more likely to be difficult and prolonged, so the last thing we want to do is to create fear around birth. Instead we need to help women to remove their fear. When it comes to birth, broadly speaking there are two groups of fears:

1. Fear of the unknown.
2. Deep-rooted emotional fear.

A fear of the unknown tends to arise from a lack of education and awareness about birth. Once a woman becomes educated, many of her fears fall by the wayside. If a woman is still fearful about birth after undertaking a reasonable level of birth education, then she most likely has the second group of fears: deep-rooted emotional fears. These fears have been formed as a result of her entire life experience from the moment she was born—her upbringing, education and her social and cultural experiences. This last aspect is perhaps the most relevant to this discussion.

Our beliefs about something like childbirth will build up over time and will come from personal conversations, interactions and experiences, and exposure to the culture around us. Today, this means what we see in our Facebook feeds, created by complex algorithms, is more likely to feed us more of what we want, rather than a balanced perspective.

It cannot be denied that there is so much about birth that makes it a perfect basis for drama: the emotion and the sheer magic and the power of birth. Unfortunately, in its most widespread form it is a drawn-out event that lasts hours if not days and takes place very slowly with often very little happening. So while we can appreciate it being the target for TV shows and films, is it any wonder that it is highly edited so that a sense of drama is created when often there isn't any?

PSYCHOLOGICAL IMPACT OF CHILDBIRTH MYTHS

Women come to me because they have fears during childbirth that they want to clear and they want help using my fear-clearance technique, the *Head Trash Clearance Method*. The *Head Trash Clearance Method* requires you to be very specific about your fears to enable you to clear them. Since I've started this work, I have been documenting the fears that many women share with me, and there is one thing that is quite striking: many of these fears can be directly linked to the childbirth myths that are sustained by the media. I'd like to dig deeper into these childbirth myths so that we can fully appreciate their psychological impact in terms of the fears they trigger amongst women.

Fear of Pain

A fear of pain is the most common fear I come across. This was my biggest fear in my first pregnancy and because of it, my birth plan early in my pregnancy was highly medicalised, including an elective C-section to avoid the "unavoidable" pain. Many women feel this way about pain and birth and hence opt for an elective C-section. Unfortunately, when it comes to pain and childbirth, there are two things that make pain worse or increase our experience or perception of it:

1. Anticipating pain.
2. Fear of pain.

When a woman believes that childbirth is painful, she will be tapping into both of these pain anxieties, which have the potential for increasing her own experience of it. She will no doubt anticipate pain because she has been led to believe *"childbirth hurts; we all know that!"*; moreover, if she's heard that it's the worst pain she will ever experience, then of course she will fear it all the more.

Fear of Losing Dignity and Respect

Women who have not undertaken any childbirth education tend to believe that they will birth on their backs; and it's not hard to imagine how vulnerable this will make them feel. Add to that the potential of having an audience of people you don't know, some of whom might be men, and you have an unpleasant combination that can easily lead to feeling of a loss of all sense of dignity and respect. Given the physical and emotional demands of labour, all these feelings will be exacerbated; and this is something that the mother-to-be is very aware of. As a woman thinks about her upcoming birth, these fears of losing dignity and respect may be very difficult to deal with, especially if the woman believes dignity and respect are all important.

Fear of Losing Control

Birth is already a vulnerable time for a woman, so when she imagines that she will need to be in a physically vulnerable position such as lying on her back, then it may well lead to her losing her sense of control. Feeling like she is in control of such an important event like birth is important for a woman. A fear of losing control is a potent fear that has many facets:

(Not) Being in Control

In reality not having control or handing over control usually applies to situations or other people. If being in control is very important for people, then when other people have control over them, they often experience stress and fear, especially if they have "control issues". I often come across this in high-achieving professional women. They are used to being in control in their work and home life, so the idea of surrendering control at such a vulnerable time as childbirth is very threatening to them. They might try to retain a sense of control through developing very detailed birth plans or giving clear instructions for their birth partners. This need for control has the potential to create unnecessary stress during birth, so I help them to lose their fear of not being in control and to become more accepting of it.

Feeling Out of Control

This is different from not being in control. This is an emotion where the person feels out of control even when that feeling doesn't necessarily have a basis in reality. We often hear people say how they felt completely out of control in a particular situation; and yet from the outside it looked like they'd had it together. If this emotional response takes hold it in fact often leads to the losing control of oneself. For many this means losing control emotionally, losing ones grip, not being able to keep it together, perhaps getting emotional or angry. But it can also mean losing control of one's body and doing things involuntarily. Birth plays directly into this fear, as women imagine that they will not be able to cope or will scream in pain, sob uncontrollably or experience bodily functions that they have no control over. All of these images are perpetuated by media representations of childbirth, so this fear is very real and plays directly into a fear of losing dignity and respect.

Pressures on Health and Social Care

New parents face a multitude of stressors—from the lack of traditional support structures and community to the rising costs of childcare and housing. If they are also dealing with extreme emotional pressures too, some people simply cannot cope, thereby putting even more strain on social care systems. Contrast that to a positive birth experience where a woman is left feeling empowered from her birth:

- The feeling of empowerment from her birth raises the confidence of a mother about her ability to parent.
- Mother and baby form a strong bond.
- The mother is able to breastfeed easily, providing her baby with essential nutrients.
- The family are able to celebrate future birthdays, because they are free of difficult memories.
- The family unit is better placed emotionally to handle the ups and downs of parenting and managing a family.

Thus there is an enormous societal benefit to promoting a positive birth, even without considering the economic benefits. Helping women to experience positive birth experiences can help to reduce health-care costs significantly.

A woman who is fearful around birth is more likely to choose a C-section, and given that a planned caesarean costs on average £2369 compared to the £1665 cost of a vaginal birth, we can already see how much fear costs the UK health-care system (Schroeder et al. 2012). It is estimated that 14% of C-sections are carried out for women who are choosing them due to anxiety. If a woman chooses to birth at home, then her birth is even cheaper still (a hospital birth costs 60% more than a home birth). Also a positive birth experience is less likely to lead to the mother experiencing postnatal depression or her husband experiencing PTSD; thus the family will require less ongoing health-care support. The National Institute for Health & Care Excellence (NICE) assessed the impact of offering UK women mental health support during their pregnancy on C-section rates and as a result are increasing spending in this area.

> I just wanted to let you know that I had a home birth which was amazing! I used all my (your) mindset skills, totally let go & his head came out in 3 pushes! There was no tearing at all. No drugs & no gas & air. All in

all, it was just amazing to have him at home. A huge thank you for your brilliant podcasts—I loved Fearless Birthing & the head trash clearance method & they definitely were amazing tools that I used to set up my birth in my head & on the day. I'm so pleased I found you!

Birth Is Not Entertainment

Our birth is a sacred event that has a far-reaching impact in our lives. One birth affects the whole family in very important ways that ripple out to the community, so it's dangerous to view it as an isolated event that can be treated lightly. The birthing moment needs to be fiercely protected. However, we find ourselves in a situation where childbirth is not being treated with the respect it deserves and where the media are relentlessly pushing consistently damaging messages. This creates a sense of fear around birth that has far-reaching impact that reaches beyond the birthing mother.

What Can We Do to Bring About Change?

While it may appear that the future of birth appears depressing, there is still opportunity to bring about positive change. The fragmentation and decentralisation of the media means that mainstream outlets such as popular TV channels, radio stations, newspapers and magazines are reaching a lower share of the audience. Contrast this with the ease with which smaller providers can publish content such as blogs, videos and podcasts. When done well, this content can attract a tribe of fans and can have a real impact on women.

I know that the media can make a difference about how women feel about birth because I'm part of it, albeit it is new media. I know my podcast is helping women to lose their fear around birth because I receive countless emails from women sharing their stories and experiences with me. Emails like this are typical:

> THANK YOU SO MUCH ALEXIA for taking the time to get the fear free birth message out there to moms! I didn't know there was any other way until finding your podcast. I was soooo afraid to even get pregnant, because I knew the baby had to come out somehow! Was SURE I'd plan a C-section/epidural… ANYTHING to keep the pain down. Though my mum had me no-drugs in a hospital in the 80s, I have been exposed

to negative birth stories my entire life. I had the phobia of childbirth! ALEXIA you SAVED ME! I am confident that I can handle it naturally (God willing!!!) and AT HOME for my first baby ... Xoxoxoxo

I wanted to thank you for taking the time to do these podcasts, I listen to them in bed every night too and your voice sends me so sleep. I now have a birth plan in place that makes me happy and I feel like a warrior woman who will be able to give birth to my son without fear!

Clearly the media contributes significantly to how women feel about birth. It might not always be part of the problem, but it can certainly be part of the solution, and that is where I believe we have a huge opportunity.

Creating new ways for women to learn about birth is one way to bring about change, but we also need to get to the root of the problem and that means tackling the mainstream media providers. This can feel like an overwhelming task when there are hundreds if not thousands of media outlets, all able to reach thousands if not millions of women. Add to that the countless journalists and reporters who each put their own spin on the content they create, and it can quickly feel like too big a task to even contemplate. But there are some obvious places to start.

Target High Profile Birth Related TV Shows

Find ways to put pressure on shows like *One Born Every Minute* to address the problems they are contributing to, either through the producers or the broadcaster.

I made an attempt at this and created a petition on change.org in 2015 for Channel 4, the UK broadcaster of *One Born Every Minute*, to portray a more balanced view of childbirth. Within three days the petition had 600 signatures from a single Facebook post. This elicited a high-profile media response that interpreted my petition as a demand to ban the show, which it wasn't. Nevertheless it instigated a worthwhile debate in the media around the role that TV shows like can have on women's view of birth and more importantly their level of fear. This culminated in a live radio debate on BBC Radio 5Live with the producers of the show in late 2015. This debate made it very clear to me that the producers don't fully understand the impact their show has. If they were educated on the far-reaching impact of their show, they may be open to making some slight changes to their programme. For example, they could include a message at the beginning of the show that makes it clear that the series is about hospital births, but that other birth options are available. Furthermore, the producers could point out that the show is edited considerably to focus on the moments that they believe we'd like to see. Additionally, a more educational and informative narrative could be adopted in parts of the show to provide context. For example, if a woman is choosing to have an epidural, then either show a nurse or midwife talking to the woman to let her know the risks and impact on her baby, or have a narrator explain this to the viewer. These are small changes that could have a positive impact while not sacrificing the entertainment value of the show.

Fund Content that Educates and Reduces Fear in Women

This can either be through a government-run campaign or a grant made available to media producers and content creators for projects that satisfy certain criteria around childbirth education and removal of fear.

Engage with Professional Associations Related to Media Production

By engaging directly with journalists, editors, scriptwriters and producers, we can help them to understand the far-reaching impact of their work beyond its mere entertainment value.

Conclusion

I agree with Prof. Dahlen's comment that "media reflects and creates reality". Unfortunately, we find ourselves in a position whereby, in the context of birth, the media tends to reflect, and therefore perpetuate, a narrow view of birth that does not necessarily support positive birth outcomes for families. The persistent nature of the dramatic and fear-based messages that women are subjected to within our culture and through the media contributes to unnecessary levels of fear around birth. I believe that we can use the media available to us to bring about positive change and instead of feeding their fears, we should be looking to educate and inspire women so that they feel empowered to choose and prepare for a positive birth experience.

Editor's Note: Leachman provided insight into some of the fears that pregnant women face during their pregnancy. She notes how lack of positive information compounds these fears, highlighting a role for midwives in demystifying birth. In Chap. 6, Rodger et al. explore further how midwives in antenatal clinics can better use waiting rooms to maximise health promotion and support women using technology throughout their pregnancy, whilst Dahlen has her own contribution in Chap. 8.

REFERENCE

Schroeder, E., S. Petrou, N. Patel, J. Hollowell, D. Puddicombe, M. Redshaw, and P. Brocklehurst. 2012. Cost effectiveness of alternative planned places of birth in woman at low risk of complications: Evidence from the Birthplace in England national prospective cohort study. *British Medical Journal,* 344. Published online: http://www.bmj.com/content/344/bmj.e2292.

CHAPTER 6

'Passing Time': A Qualitative Study of Health Promotion Practices in an Antenatal Clinic Waiting Room

Dianne Rodger, Andrew Skuse and Michael Wilmore

Abstract The authors explore the information needs and preferences of pregnant women through a study of health-promotion strategies employed in an antenatal clinic waiting room at a tertiary hospital in the Northern suburbs of Adelaide, Australia. Conducted as part of a wider health communication project ('Health-e Baby'), the chapter provides a detailed assessment of how these spaces are used by staff to convey health messages related to pregnancy and how pregnant women interacted with these materials whilst waiting for their appointments. Rodger, Skuse and Wilmore's observational data is complimented by data drawn from semi-structured interviews (n = 35), which enables

D. Rodger (✉) · A. Skuse
University of Adelaide, Adelaide, SA, Australia
e-mail: dianne.rodger@adelaide.edu.au

A. Skuse
e-mail: andrew.skuse@adelaide.edu.au

M. Wilmore
Bournemouth University, Bournemouth, UK
e-mail: mwilmore@bournemouth.ac.uk

© The Author(s) 2017
A. Luce et al. (eds.), *Midwifery, Childbirth and the Media*,
DOI 10.1007/978-3-319-63513-2_6

them to explore how waiting rooms can be used to maximise the potential efficacy of health promotion interventions at these important sites of interaction with antenatal patients. Preliminary insights from this chapter challenge assumptions about the efficacy of current uses of antenatal waiting rooms as a setting for the communication of health information.

Keywords Health promotion · Information · Pregnant women Waiting room · Health-e baby

Introduction

This chapter examines health-promotion strategies employed in an antenatal clinic waiting room at a tertiary hospital in the northern suburbs of Adelaide, Australia. Research was conducted as part of a wider health communication project ('Health-e Baby') that explored the information needs and preferences of pregnant women. While the waiting room context was not the sole or central focus of this study, the project included periods of observation conducted in the waiting room. This allowed us to assess (i) how this space was used by staff to convey health messages related to pregnancy, (ii) how pregnant women interacted with these materials and more broadly (iii) how they used the space whilst waiting for their appointments. Observational data was complemented with data drawn from semi-structured interviews (n = 35). In this chapter we utilise these data to explore how the waiting room can best be employed in order to maximise its health-promotion potential. In turn, our preliminary insights test assumptions concerning the efficacy of antenatal waiting rooms as a key setting for the communication of health information.

Literature Review

We were unable to locate any studies that examined the effectiveness of health-promotion strategies in antenatal clinic waiting rooms. A small number of studies have analysed the provision of dedicated clinics for different cohorts of pregnant women (Jackson et al. 2006; Das et al. 2007; Hauck et al. 2013). These studies do not include detailed accounts of the nature of the clinic space (i.e., size, layout) or the role of waiting room education in their analysis of any reported impacts. Hauck et al.'s (2013) study illustrates that women who attended a dedicated childbirth and mental illness clinic understood the clinic as a safe and secure place that enabled them to build relationships of trust with a small number of staff, free from stigma. However, they do not examine if or how the physical features of the clinic may have contributed to these understandings. Kildea et al. (2012) study of an Aboriginal and Torres Strait Islander antenatal clinic is an important contribution to the literature because it does consider both the location of the clinic and the physical layout of the clinic. Their study found that a lack of privacy and overcrowding in the clinic made it difficult for staff to discuss sensitive issues with pregnant women and to build rapport and trust. Furthermore, the waiting room was described by women as an unappealing space that their partners did not want to use (Kildea et al. 2012, p. 8). Kildea's study illustrates the value of examining the physical geography of waiting rooms and how they are used by pregnant women, their partners and families.

More broadly, there is sparse literature examining the value of waiting rooms as spaces for health education. Leong and Horn (2014, p. 145) note the paucity of research about how these spaces might be better utilised for health promotion (i.e., how resources in the waiting room like posters and pamphlets can best be utilised to enable 'people to increase control over, and to improve, their health' (World Health Organisation, The Ottawa Charter for Health Promotion 1986). Similarly, McGrath and Tempier (2003) question the effectiveness of the waiting room as an educational space. They argue that until more is known about the 'culture of the waiting room', including the factors that might influence patient's likeliness to read or take health promotion materials, health professionals should give patients health information directly to ensure minimum standards of communication and information provision between health professionals and patients (McGrath and Tempier 2003, p. 1043). Several studies have focused on the impact of individual health promotion strategies utilised in waiting rooms, including posters and noticeboards (Ward and Hawthorn 1994; Wicke et al. 1994; Montazeri and Sajadian 2004; Ashe et al. 2006) and closed circuit television programs (Cockington 1995), but these have not utilised a holistic approach to consider how different health promotion elements (i.e., leaflets, posters, television programs) are utilised by patients.

Health promotion practitioners have long-understood that using multiple communication channels to promote consistent and relevant messages has the best potential to promote knowledge acquisition, increased confidence, lower anxiety or behaviour change (UNICEF 2006). Studies of multi-channel/method promotion strategies have tended to use quantitative approaches that rely on self-reporting (Bamgboye and Jarallah 1994; Ajayi 2002). These studies provide important information about the media preferences of patients but are limited by a lack of contextual data. Gignon et al. (2012) provide valuable insights into how general practitioners (GPs) choose the media displayed in waiting rooms, but do not examine how they are understood and used by patients themselves. Leong and Horn's (2014) observational study of waiting areas in two North American sickle cell disease treatment clinics corrects this failing. Their work illustrates how participant observation provides a detailed understanding of the design of the health promotion strategies used in waiting rooms. They found that of the roughly 500 people observed during their study less than 10 read books, magazines or newspapers and all of them brought these with them. This contrasted with high levels of digital media use, with one in two people using mobile technology to pass the time. These findings informed the design of a health 'station' to be used in sickle cell clinic waiting rooms comprised of an information poster, tablet-based app (software application) and two models of blood cells made from fabric. Although user testing found that some groups had difficulty utilising the educational materials, overall there was a marked increase in patients' engagement with the provided resources. Leong and Horn's (2014) work highlights the value of paying close attention to what people actually do in waiting rooms in order to consider the 'real world applicability' of health-promotion interventions (Leong and Horn 2014, p. 153).

Methods

Five hours of participant observation was conducted in the waiting room of the family clinic at the study hospital. The family clinic at the study hospital, henceforth referred to as the clinic, fulfils a range of functions, including paediatric, gynaecological, antenatal and postnatal health care.

During these periods of observation, the first author sat in the waiting room with a clipboard and, following Madden (2010, p. 123), wrote scratch notes that documented the layout of the space, the health-promotion strategies utilised in the space and how patients and staff utilised the space. While detailed notes regarding the readability, design and layout of posters displayed in the waiting room were taken, no formal content analysis tools were used to systematically assess the posters; and this represents a modest limitation of the study that is tempered by the low levels of print material usage witnessed during periods of observation. Different seating positions within the space were chosen during the observation period to enable the researcher to document any variations in patient behaviour based on clinic layout. The presence of a researcher in the waiting room was discrete and did not appear to unduly affect the 'waiting' behaviour of patients. Formal observations were conducted in five separate one-hour blocks over the course of two weeks. Observation was conducted on different days and in both the morning and afternoon. Immediately after each observation period the scratch notes were consolidated into field notes, which were longer form, narrative accounts (Madden 2010, p. 125). The low number of hours spent conducting participant observation and the ad hoc nature of the selection of times/days is a limitation of this study.[1] We recommend that further work conducted in this area should entail full days of participant observation or at minimum, longer sessions of 2–3 hours over a lengthier period of time.

Semi-structured interviews were also conducted with pregnant women (n = 35) on-site at the study hospital in a private interview room.[2] Women were recruited face-to-face by the project's Research Midwife and Midwives working in the antenatal clinic. As we discuss elsewhere (Rodger et al. 2013), this convenience sample was a limitation of the study. Women answered questions about their access to and use of different media, their information-seeking habits relating to pregnancy and their views about the communication practices employed at the study hospital, including the waiting room. Semi-structured interviews were chosen to enable the researchers to leverage the strengths of both structured and un-structured interviews, namely, the ability to incorporate both fixed, pre-determined questions and to allow space for free-flowing exchanges (O'Reilly 2009, p. 126). An interview schedule was developed by the first author in collaboration with the research team.[3]

Analysis

Field notes describing patient and staff behaviour in the waiting room and women's own accounts of their experience in the waiting room were valuable sources of data that were analysed in this study. Field notes and interview transcriptions were analysed using 'ethnographic analysis' (O'Reily 2012) by the first author to identify material relevant to the aim of the study, namely, the suitability and effectiveness of the waiting room as a channel of health promotion. This process is described by O'Reilly (2012, p. 186) as 'making sense of it all', a phrase which she notes is intentionally vague because analysis in ethnographic research is not a discrete activity but is closely connected to data collection. Whilst O'Reilly (2012, pp. 186, 187) stresses the iterative-inductive nature of ethnographic research and the constant thinking and analysis that takes place during research itself, she argues that there is an identifiable 'sorting' phase of analysis where field notes and interview transcripts are re-ordered into categories. In this chapter the reordering of the data into categories was conducted by the first author, who was more intimately familiar with the total data set (Morse 2015, p. 1218). These categories were then discussed with the co-authors and developed into the themes discussed in this chapter.

Clinic Context

The clinic at the study hospital is open from 8:30 a.m. to 5:00 p.m., five days a week (Monday to Friday) and is the location for the first antenatal appointment of a pregnancy, referred to by staff as a 'triage' appointment. Staff in the clinic also provide antenatal care beyond the first appointment, depending on judgments made about the patients' level of 'risk' and care requirements. The clinic space is an irregular shape with very few straight walls or right-angle corners. This is important because women's experience of the space differs depending on where they elect to sit (women are given a number when they report to the front desk and can choose their own seat). The layout also means that there is no central focal point to be utilised when attempting to communicate health messages. A large reception/midwives' station is located in the approximate centre of the space. The reception/midwives station is surrounded on three sides by waiting areas that are separated by pathways. Each of these areas contains individual chairs that are arranged in rows. One of these areas is a space with toys and books that is provided for clients with children. There are no health-promotion materials on the walls in this section. A rotating information stand is located in this area and primarily features health materials relating to childrearing. The second waiting area is located directly in front of the reception station. This area is bound on one side by a large glass window. A small table, pinboard and rotating information stand occupy the far corner of this area. The third waiting area is located on the left-hand side of the reception station. This area has the largest expanse of wall space and the highest concentration of posters. This use of large posters, as well as the provision of a variety of pamphlets via information stands is the central health-promotion strategy employed in the clinic.

This description of the waiting room, while capturing a sense of its spatial orientation and the health-promotion strategies employed therein, does not capture the hive of activity that occurs in the pursuit of passing time. During the observation period we documented a diverse range of behaviours, including toddlers crawling underneath chairs and being reprimanded by frustrated parents, women bickering with reception staff, numerous people closely examining content on their mobile phones or talking on their phones, people reading magazines like *Marie Claire* or simply sitting patiently and waiting. While this account of 'waiting practice' highlights a variety of different activities, our observational and qualitative data reveal a range of dominant practices. These include (i) mobile phone use; (ii) talking with partners, friends or family members; (iii) sitting and observing the surroundings; (iv) reading one's own or provided literature such as magazines or books; and (v) parenting young children.

Some of these activities are social and some are individual, but most are undertaken simply in order to pass time. It is in this context that multiple health-promotion strategies are employed. Paying attention to these social and inherently qualitative details is important because they help to highlight both the agency and diversity of the waiting room 'audience'. In turn, such data illustrate that it is dangerous to assume that patients occupying waiting rooms are actively interested in engaging with the health information provided while they wait. Indeed, observation confirms that many women and their partners, friends or family members are relatively disengaged from their immediate environment. Interviews suggested that women viewed the waiting room as a transitory space where they would wait *before* receiving health information (i.e., in their appointments) not a space *for* health information. Waiting for an appointment was understood to be a dull task, and women sought out entertainment to avoid boredom. Yet, as we discuss below, women typically utilised their own means (mobile phones, talking to partners, books) to fulfil these needs and not health-promotion materials provided in the waiting room. In the following section we outline how women responded to two key health-promotion strategies utilised by the hospital (posters and pamphlets). We then discuss a number of broader mitigating factors that shaped their receptiveness to health communication in the waiting room.

Existing Approaches: Posters and Pamphlets

Several posters adorn the walls of the clinic waiting room. Some of these are posters produced by state and federal Australian government organisations, while others have been designed and compiled by clinic staff members. As such, the design quality and readability of the posters varies dramatically. Participants were asked if they had looked at any of the posters displayed in the waiting room. Of these, 81% said yes, suggesting that most women were aware of the posters and had engaged with them to some extent. Yet, when asked further questions about the posters that they had viewed women often found it difficult to provide specific details, suggesting that their engagement was fleeting:

> I did actually [look at the posters], but I can't remember what I was actually looking at, but something about twins...I think maybe postnatal depression was there, I can't remember the rest. (Nora, 29)

Similarly, when asked if they had 'learnt' anything from the posters displayed in the waiting room, women often found it difficult to identify any of the key messages associated with them. Dawn (a 29-year-old) was able to name a number of the posters on display, but when asked what she learnt from the posters she replied, 'Nothing. They were just there. Too far away to take in'. Another participant reported that she had not read any of the posters in the clinic and that it was difficult to do so unless you were very close to them (Ingrid, 33). During the observation period we did not see anyone walking up to a poster to examine it in more detail. This suggests that while people may look at a poster's main heading, which is usually written in a large font and can be read from a distance, they are less likely to read the smaller supporting text associated with it. This observation was confirmed in interviews, with some women indicating that the font size of some posters needed to be larger if they were to take anything meaningful from them. In this respect, the fragmented layout of the clinic makes it difficult for waiting patients to interact with health-promotion materials. Patient distance from posters, poor design and the fact that they could not be viewed from all areas significantly reduced their effectiveness. When asked if she had viewed any posters in the clinic waiting room, 40-year-old Casey noted, 'Actually no, I've kept thinking that next time I come in I'll sit round the other side where the posters are'. It was unclear from this statement whether Casey intended to switch seats in order to engage with the posters or to have something entertaining on the wall to look at.

Posters stand in relationship to another body of print material available in the waiting room, namely, pamphlets. The clinic waiting room contains information stands displaying approximately 30 pamphlets. The vast majority of these differ from the materials that are provided at the first antenatal appointment, although a few are duplicates (i.e., provided at the first appointment *and* available in the waiting room). A number of available pamphlets advertise a range of support services, while the majority support an explicit behaviour change or educational goal (i.e., breastfeeding, safe sleeping, postnatal depression/mental health). While we observed one woman reading a parenting magazine taken from a nearby coffee table and one woman turning the information stands and looking at the pamphlet titles, we did not see anyone take a pamphlet from the waiting room. Interviews confirmed that a low number of women took printed material from the waiting room. Of the 32 women who were asked about the waiting room pamphlets, 6 reported taking one away, 2 looked at pamphlets but did not keep them, and 24 did not engage with them in any way. This number included 3 women that were completely unaware that they were even available in the waiting room.

Interview and observational data confirm that the print material provided in the clinic waiting room is used infrequently. However, the provision of such material is deemed important by patients and health staff in case additional information is being sought. The specialised nature of these pamphlets means that they will not appeal to all women and the strategy is a low-cost solution to potential information needs. Nonetheless, far greater attention could be paid to their placement and presentation in order to promote additional usage. For example, one participant stated that it would be helpful if there was a prominent 'wall' of pamphlets that would be easier to view. Other women incorrectly assumed that the available print material would be the same as those given to them by midwives at their initial antenatal appointment (Wilmore et al. 2015). When asked if she took any pamphlets from the waiting room, 23-year-old Melanie stated, 'No cos' [sic] they all get given to you'. Thinking through how print resources are used within spaces such as the clinic is important to increasing their relevance and use. While we identified low usage rates this does not mean that such resources are irrelevant to all patients. However, it does suggest that greater attention needs to be paid to prioritising key messages within the clinic space and serious consideration needs to be given to how posters and other print materials relate to each other. Our study suggests that the print-based approach in the clinic struggles to make an impact. In the following section we argue that health promoters seeking to utilise the waiting room as an educational space need to be attentive to a number of factors, including the length of wait times, competing interests that complicate the idea of a receptive audience, patient information needs and preferences and their mobile phone use.

Waiting Time

The effectiveness of waiting rooms as a place where health communication can occur is to an extent mitigated by the length of the wait. Too short a wait and there is little opportunity for health communication to occur. Too long, and boredom can give way to personal strategies focused on entertainment, such as reading and mobile phone use. Waiting times within the clinic varied widely. Some patients did not wait long for their appointments (1–10 minutes), particularly if their appointment was with a midwife, rather than a doctor. These patients had little time to engage with posters or look at the other forms of health communication. Other patients had far longer waiting times and while deducing an average wait time is beyond the scope of this paper, it was common for patients to wait up to 30 minutes, especially to see a doctor. Still, these are relatively low wait times that differ significantly from two studies of waiting room behaviour, which reported mean wait times of 148 minutes (Bamgboye and Jarallah 1994) and 144 minutes (Ajayi 2002). These short wait times of up to 30 minutes did impact on women's utilisation of the health-promotion material displayed in the waiting room: 'You're called in pretty quickly' (Belinda, 33) and 'I was only waiting for about 2 minutes' (Alison, 26). In a context where waiting times can be relatively short, a health-promotion strategy that prioritises a few key messages and supporting materials is potentially a preferable option. While patients cite short wait times, observational data highlights that longer wait times do not necessarily lead to engagement with the education materials provided in the clinic waiting room. Therefore, health-promotion strategies need to consider the relative waiting times of patients and tailor strategies and approaches that are capable of making an impact, such as promoting a modest number of key health messages that can be easily appropriated. Irrespective of wait time, it is also important to consider that the waiting room was also understood by our participants as a space of competing interests and distractions that were not always conducive to health education.

Competing Interests

The need to complete tasks such as filling in paperwork were factors that limited women's ability to engage with the provided health-promotion materials. For example, 19-year-old Bernadette stated that she was too busy filling out forms to concentrate on the posters displayed in the waiting room. Others reported that they were too preoccupied by caring responsibilities to engage with educational materials. Jackie, a mother of four children, stated that she was distracted in the waiting room 'with a two-year-old running around' (Jackie, 39). In addition to obligations such as monitoring children and filling out paperwork, pregnant women frequently opted to use their wait time to engage with their own media, most commonly mobile phones, which are discussed in detail below. Our analysis highlights that many women utilising the waiting room were indifferent to the range of print materials being offered; and while this indifference has been shown to sometimes reflect a misplaced perception that this information offered has been previously provided, it also suggests alternative strategies are being employed to address perceived information needs.

Information Needs and Preferences

Women's individual information needs and preferences were found to play a key role in determining the modest use of the health-promotion resources made available in the waiting room. Pauline, a 27-year-old woman, stated she 'stared out the window' while she waited for her antenatal appointment and did not look at any of the posters. She said that she did not interact with the posters because—

> I'd already pretty much looked up everything I wanted to know [before the first appointment] and I figured talking to the Midwife was going to be the best.

Likewise, Jane reported that she would prefer to search for information using a search engine on her phone or to ask a health professional in person rather than 'flick through a brochure' (Jane, 21). This echoes the wider use of mobile phones by patients within the waiting room identified through observation. In addition to the information medium, the content of some of the health media provided in the waiting room did not resonate with some of our participants. Gwen indicated that the content of many of the posters was not relevant to her, in particular identifying posters that promoted smoking cessation or those that targeted Aboriginal and Torres Strait Islander peoples. Nonetheless, she concluded that the posters would be helpful for other women in the hospital's catchment area:

> I think that they serve their purpose for what they're trying to get out there...like I said I think they're area appropriate so, to the demographic around here. (Gwen, 32)

Household structure and previous pregnancy experience were two important factors that influenced women's information needs, with some women stating that they did not engage with the health-promotion material in the waiting room because they were from a large family with many children or because they had previously been pregnant, which implies experience and a lack of need for further information. When asked what she did while waiting for her appointment, 23-year-old Melanie said, 'Um, not much cos' [sic] I've been pregnant before' (Melanie, 23). Hailey indicated that she did not read any posters because she had played a role in raising her siblings and had intergenerational childrearing experience. Elliot chose not to consult posters because 'I've done this [pregnancy] four times so I sort of know all the information' (Elliot, 25). Our analysis shows that while some women reject the need for further 'education' due to their relative experience, others display clear preferences over their choice of communications medium and types of media content with which they engage. These preferences are not currently addressed within existing waiting room health-promotion strategies.

Mobile Phones

People waiting within the clinic are not required to turn off their mobile phones; and while they wait, many people use them to play games, read text messages and make voice calls. When asked what they did in the waiting room, six women discussed their mobile phone use without prompting. Responses included answers like 'Turn on my phone' (Frances, 24), 'I've got the phone 24/7' (Kelly, 19), '[I] got out my phone' (Casey, 40) and 'I just wait, I've got my phone apps' (Yasmin, 23).[4] Observational data adds further weight to this finding, with numerous examples of pregnant women and their partners or family members using information communication technologies as a means of passing their waiting time. Indeed, on more than one occasion people who came into the waiting room together would each use their phones individually while sitting next to each other. This supports Leong and Horn's (2014, p. 148) contention that the high levels of technology use (i.e., smart phones, tablets) in contemporary waiting rooms represents an opportunity for health promotion, one that continues to be missed for want of recognising the realities of contemporary mobile media use occurring within the waiting room space.

Beyond the confines of the waiting room, our quantitative data reveals that 97% of women regularly accessed social media, predominantly using their mobile phone as the primary source of access to Internet-based media and information. Furthermore, 89% of our cohort had used an internet-based search to locate pregnancy-related health information, with many women indicating that the internet would be the first source that they would consult if they had a question about their pregnancy. Yet, despite these high usage levels, the women interviewed were found to be relatively poor at distinguishing between high- and low-quality health-information sources. Others felt overwhelmed by the amount of available health information and wanted to be directed to information sources that they knew they could trust (See Rodger et al. [2013] for further discussion). Importantly, high levels of trust were placed in the study hospital and these data point to an approach that may yield greater impact in terms of electronically mediated health-promotion strategies undertaken within the waiting room space. Increasingly, the availability of wireless networks is enabling institutions such as hospitals to offer access to the internet, and specifically, to relevant health-related sites (Ngoc 2008). Enabling patients to pass their waiting time by engaging with sites or 'apps' that are 'pushed' to users and effectively 'certified' by trusted health institution is one approach that may yield greater impact than current paper-based health-promotion strategies.

Yet, as de la Vega and Miro (2014) note, there is a large gap between commercial health apps and the scientific health literature. De la Vega and Miro found that while there are a growing number of peer-reviewed studies of scientifically supported, evidence-based health applications, very few of these apps are available to the general public. Conversely, commercial apps that are readily accessible in app stores frequently lack scientific validation. This suggests that health providers could play a key role in distributing trusted health apps. Similarly, in their study of pregnant women's use of smartphone applications and Internet resources, Kraschnewski et al. (2014) found that health providers need to better support women to utilise these technologies to access pregnancy-related information. Free downloads of pregnancy apps in waiting rooms would enable patients to avoid download costs and to take away a bank of information for use beyond the confines of this specific setting. Recognising the potential of contemporary mobile phone use, when ownership is near universal, is important to health-promotion strategies' being dragged into the twenty-first century. A strategy that understands the way in which patients use the waiting room space is critical to developing health communication materials and approaches that are informed by evidence.

Conclusion: Rethinking the Waiting Room and Enhancing Health Promotion

The previous analysis of information needs and preferences, 'waiting practices' and of existing health-promotion strategies adopted in the clinic waiting room points to an approach that is hopeful, rather than evidence-based and tailored. The low cost, but low impact, print-dominated strategy employed in the waiting room runs counter to the dominant media/technology use reported by patients in interviews and reinforced by observational data. The inability to target mobile phone users is perhaps the most obvious shortcoming of the existing health communication and promotion approach utilised within the clinic.

While the waiting room space is one that is closely associated with opportunities to impart information and promote health, our study reveals that little attention is paid by health promoters to how patients utilise the waiting room space. Our research found that pregnant women found different ways to occupy their time while they waited and that these waiting strategies did not frequently involve interacting with the health-promotion materials or information provided by the hospital. Women tended to seek out their own entertainment and spent their waiting time engaged in activities such as talking to their partner or family members, using their mobile phones, reading novels or parenting their children. These activities coupled with short wait-times limited women's exposure to and engagement with health-promotion material. These findings complicate the idea that patients in waiting rooms are captive audiences who are potentially receptive to enhancing their health literacies while they wait. While it is tempting to view time spent in a waiting room as an opportunity for education, our research suggests that pregnant women have their own strategies and preferences for how this time is passed, and these are predominantly focused on being entertained. This leads us to an important finding, namely, that if health-promotion initiatives designed for waiting rooms are to be successful they must be able to quickly attract the attention of the waiting audience and cut through a multitude of technological and social distractions.

This finding has implications for the type of health promotion undertaken, the communication channels and approaches that are utilised within such spaces as well as the relative value of contemporary print driven strategies. Evidence suggests that while print-based strategies may periodically capture the attention of a waiting patient and are undoubtedly cheap to undertake, often such material is ignored in favour of activities such as mobile phone use. These findings suggest that significant opportunities to promote better health are being missed, opportunities that rest with increasing personal access to and use of internet capable mobile phones within spaces such as hospital waiting rooms. The potential to harness free-to-access wireless networks to promote trusted and relevant internet-based health information sources or to 'push' relevant health applications provides an opportunity to actively 'disrupt' patients' waiting time and harness a technology with which they are already engaged. Contemporary communication preferences suggest that patients actively search out health information using simple web-based searches and increasingly via health apps (Rodger et al. 2013). In turn, this suggests that there is considerable health-promotion and behaviour-change potential in adopting a more forward-looking health-promotion strategy that incorporates popular mobile technology use and is more squarely built on an understanding of what patients do as they 'pass time' in the waiting room.

Editor's Note: Rodger et al. pointed out in this chapter that traditional methods of engaging pregnant women in waiting rooms needs to change. Midwives need to engage women via health apps and harness technology to engage women in the online environments they are already inhabiting. This will help women to differentiate between good and poor information. In the next chapter, we examine midwives' perspectives on engaging with media, highlighting three themes around changing discourse, using social media in day-to-day work and media training for midwives.

Notes

1. The central aim of this study was to explore how women used information and communication technologies to access health information during pregnancy. As part of this project, we considered women's access to and use of other pregnancy-related information sources, including material provided in the waiting room. However, funding priorities meant that this aspect of the study was not the main concern.
2. This research conformed to the 'Statement on Human Experimentation' by the National Health and Medical Research Council of Australia and was approved by the Adelaide Health Service Human Research Ethics Committee (HREC 2011026). All subjects gave written informed consent and are referred to by pseudonyms throughout.
3. Individual client interviews were typically one hour in duration and were audio-recorded and then transcribed by the first author or the research midwife. All women quoted in this paper were pregnant at the time of interview with varying gestational ages from 11 to 37 weeks. The mean gestational age at point of interview was 15.7 weeks.
4. Whilst it could be hypothesised that younger women would be more likely to use a mobile phone, our study included women aged 18–40 (median age 28), all of whom had a mobile phone, with the exception of one woman who was sharing her partner's phone at the time of the interview. The use of mobile phone functions like social media and internet-searching did differ from woman to woman—but we did not identify any clear correlations between age and mobile phone preferences.

Acknowledgments We acknowledge the Australian Research Council and SA Health, who provided the funding for this research through a Linkage Grant (LP110100405) and the members of the Health-e Baby team (Dr. Sal Humphreys, A/Prof Vicki Clifton and Research Midwife Julia Dalton). We thank the staff and women at the study hospital for their support.

References

Ajayi, I.O. 2002. Patients' waiting time at an outpatient clinic in Nigeria—can it be put to better use? *Patient Education and Counseling* 47: 121–126.
Ashe, D., P.A. Patrick, M.M. Stempel, Q. Shi, and D.A. Brand. 2006. Educational posters to reduce antibiotic use. *Pediatric Health Care* 20 (3): 192–197.
Bamgboye, E.A., and J.S. Jarallah. 1994. Long-waiting outpatients: Target audience for health education. *Patient Education and Counseling* 23 (1): 49–54.
Cockington, R.A. 1995. Health promotion using television in hospital waiting rooms: The Adelaide children's parent education project. *Journal of Paediatrics and Child Health* 31 (6): 523–526.
Das, S., J.S. Dhulkotia, J. Brook, and O. Amu. 2007. The impact of a dedicated antenatal clinic on the obstetric and neonatal outcomes in adolescent pregnant women. *Journal of Obstetrics and Gynaecology* 27 (5): 464–466.
de la Vega, R., and J. Miro. 2014. mHealth: A strategic field without a solid scientific soul. A systematic review of pain-related apps. *PLoS ONE* 9 (7): e101312.
Gignon, M., H. Idris, C. Manaouil, and O. Ganry. 2012. The waiting room: Vector for health education? The general practitioner's point of view. *BMC Research Notes* 5: 511.
Hauck, Y., S. Allen, F. Ronchi, D. Faulkner, J. Frayne, and T. Nguyen. 2013. Pregnancy experiences of Western Australian women attending a specialist childbirth and mental illness antenatal clinic. *Health Care for Women International* 34 (5): 380–394.
Jackson, C.J., P. Bosio, M. Habiba, J. Waugh, P. Kamal, and M. Dixon-Woods. 2006. Referral and attendance at a specialist antenatal clinic: Qualitative study of women's views. *BJOG* 113 (8): 909–913.
Kildea, S., H. Stapleton, R. Murphy, N.B. Low, and K. Gibbons. 2012. The Murri clinic: A comparative retrospective study of an antenatal clinic developed for Aboriginal and Torres Strait Islander women. *BMC Pregnancy and Childbirth* 12: 1–11.
Kraschnewski, J.L., C.H. Chuang, E.S. Poole, T. Peyton, I. Blubaugh, J. Pauli, et al. 2014. Paging "Dr. Google": Does technology fill the gap created by the prenatal care visit structure? Qualitative focus group study with pregnant women. *Journal of Medical Internet Research* 16 (6): e147.
Leong, Z.A., and M.S. Horn. 2014. Waiting for learning: Designing interactive educational materials for patient waiting areas. In *Proceedings of the 2014 conference on interaction design and children*, 145–153. Aarhus, Denmark.
Madden, R. 2010. *Being ethnographic: A guide to the theory and practice of ethnography*. Los Angeles: Sage.

McGrath, B.M., and R.P. Tempier. 2003. Is the waiting room a classroom? *Psychiatric Services* 54 (7): 1043.

Montazeri, A., and A. Sajadian. 2004. Do women read poster displays on breast cancer in waiting rooms? *Journal of Public Health* 26 (4): 355–358.

Morse, J.M. 2015. Critical analysis of strategies for determining rigor in qualitative inquiry. *Qualitative Health Research* 25 (9): 1212–1222.

Ngoc, T.V. 2008. Medical applications of wireless networks. Retrieved from http://www.cse.wustl.edu/~jain/cse574-08/ftp/medical/.

O'Reilly, K. 2009. *Key concepts in ethnography*. Los Angeles: Sage.

O'Reilly, K. 2012. *Ethnographic methods*, 2nd ed. London: Routledge.

Rodger, D., A. Skuse, M. Wilmore, S. Humphreys, J. Dalton, M. Flabouris, and V.L. Clifton. 2013. Pregnant women's use of information and communications technologies to access pregnancy-related health information in South Australia. *Australian Journal of Primary Health* 19 (4): 308–312.

Ward, K., and K. Hawthorne. 1994. Do patients read health promotion posters in the waiting room? A study in one general practice. *British Journal of General Practice* 44: 583–585.

Wicke, D.M., R.E. Lorge, R.J. Coppin, and K.P. Jones. 1994. The effectiveness of waiting room notice-boards as a vehicle for health-education. *Family Practice* 11 (3): 292–295.

Wilmore, M., D. Rodger, S. Humphreys, V.L. Clifton, J. Dalton, M. Flabouris, and A. Skuse. 2015. How midwives tailor health information materials used in antenatal care. *Midwifery* 31 (1): 74–76.

World Health Organisation. 1986. The Ottawa Charter for health promotion. Retrieved from http://www.who.int/healthpromotion/conferences/previous/ottawa/en/. Accessed 09 Feb 2017.

UNICEF. 2006. Behaviour change communication in emergencies: A toolkit. Retrieved from http://www.unicef.org/rosa/Behaviour.pdf. Accessed 09 Feb 2017.

CHAPTER 7

Midwives' Engagement with the Media

Ann Luce, Vanora Hundley, Edwin van Teijlingen, Sian Ridden and Sofie Edlund

Abstract Historically, women have learned about childbirth from their mothers and sisters, and from seeing childbirth in the family or community. In the more recent past, women would have gone to books for advice. Today, we see that women are turning to media to learn about what the experience of childbirth is like. This poses an interesting dilemma for midwives who support mothers during their pregnancy. This chapter will discuss the findings from two closely linked research projects that speak to midwives about their experience with women who are allegedly influenced by the media in their decisions about childbirth.

A. Luce (✉) · V. Hundley · E. van Teijlingen · S. Ridden · S. Edlund
Bournemouth University, Poole, UK
e-mail: aluce@bournemouth.ac.uk

V. Hundley
e-mail: vhundley@bournemouth.ac.uk

E. van Teijlingen
e-mail: evteijlingen@bournemouth.ac.uk

S. Ridden
e-mail: sianridden@hotmail.com

S. Edlund
e-mail: sofieedlund@live.se

© The Author(s) 2017
A. Luce et al. (eds.), *Midwifery, Childbirth and the Media*,
DOI 10.1007/978-3-319-63513-2_7

The chapter will explore how midwives understand their profession to be depicted in the media and will also explore how midwives engage with the media. We will provide some suggestions for midwives moving forward who wish to create more positive representations of childbirth and early labour in the media.

Keywords Midwives · Media · Fear · Media training · Social media

Traditionally, midwives have referred to fear as being a reason for rising rates of intervention in childbirth, and they put the blame for this squarely at the door of the media (Hundley et al. 2015). This fear, however, has always been portrayed as a pregnant woman's fear, not midwives' own fear. In 2014, Dahlen and Caplice published a seminal piece of research conducted in Australia and New Zealand on the fears of maternity-care providers and how their fears might impact on the women they care for. In that study, maternity-care providers indicated fears that ranged from the death of a baby, to causing harm, to losing passion or confidence in normal birth. Dahlen and Caplice (2014) did not find that 'fear of the media' ranked high on midwives' list of fears. In fact, it was nowhere to be found. Yet, it is clear from the guidance provided by professional and regulatory bodies as well as the academic literature that midwives and academics who study midwifery do fear the media, especially social media (RCM 2014; NMC 2016). These professionals are anxious about how the media portray issues, and are equally worried about their own engagement with different social media platforms and the impact either of these can have on pregnant women.

We know from research that portrayals of childbearing, and in particular of birth, both on television and in newspapers, are largely unrealistic, focusing on dramatic and risky events rather than normal birth (MacLean 2014; Luce et al. 2016). It is widely believed that these portrayals have a significant effect on women's perceptions of the birth process, influencing their behaviour towards childbirth (e.g., increasing requests for interventions such as caesarean section). Previous chapters indicate there is little evidence to support a direct link between media reports and behavioural change; the fact remains that for many women the media is an important source of information about pregnancy, birth and the postnatal period. Indeed, some reports suggest that the media has replaced antenatal education as the main source of information about childbirth (Declercq et al. 2006). But could midwives' own fears around the media impact on pregnant women? Media colleagues have suggested that midwives' failure to engage with the media has in part allowed the growth in misrepresentations around birth (Hundley et al. 2014). According to Dahlen and Caplice, 'the limited literature available about how health care provider's fears can impact women and childbirth suggests there could be a link' (2014: 266).

Historically, women have learnt about childbirth from their mothers and sisters, and from being present at the birth of a family member. Childbirth was 'women's business', and women would have had the opportunity to witness birth by assisting others in the community (Donnison 1977). However, societal changes beginning in the late nineteenth century and culminating in government recommendations for the total hospitalisation of birth in 1970 (DH, Peel Report 1970) saw the place of birth move from the community to hospital, and in many Western countries birth now occurs 'behind closed doors'. Clement (1997) was one of the first to examine the role of the media in relation to childbirth and noted that for many women television or film was the only opportunity that they had to view a birth before experiencing it for themselves. The idea that the media plays an important role in informing women about birth poses an interesting dilemma for midwives. There is a clear need for more realistic depictions of childbirth, but the key question is, Whose responsibility is it?

There has been significant debate about where the responsibility for balanced health reporting lies (Schwitzer et al. 2005; Hundley et al. 2014). In some sensitive areas, such as suicide and domestic violence, guidelines have been drawn up to assist the media in reporting these topics in a considerate and responsible manner (WHO and IASP 2008/2017; Riddoch and Orr, n.d.). Responsible reporting requires that journalists have access to a source of accurate information about the topic and therefore they argue that health professionals have a duty to engage with the media in order to make this information available (Hundley et al. 2014). United Kingdom midwives are generally reticent about engaging with the media. Indeed, warnings from employers and professional bodies have on the whole tended to discourage such activity (RCM 2014). The Nursing and Midwifery Council's guidance for nurses and midwives on social media and social networking is intended to offer a balanced view while maintaining that nurses and midwives should at all times uphold the Code (NMC 2016). However, fear of engaging with the media may be fueled by the fact that a number of National Health Service (NHS) Trusts have taken action against staff for improper use of social media (Laja 2011) and cautionary stories are cited in professional learning packages (RCM 2014). If midwives are to have a role in changing the narrative around childbirth then there is a need to understand how they perceive media discourse and how it impacts on their day-to-day work with pregnant women, as well as their own concerns and potential fears about engaging with media producers. With this in mind we conducted a qualitative study to explore midwives' experiences of media's representation of childbirth, and their views of engaging with the media.

Our in-depth interviews with a small group of midwives, working in a variety of settings (the NHS, independent practice and higher education) revealed three themes: (1) midwives engaging with media to change discourse, (2) midwives' use of social media in their day-to-day work and (3) midwives and media training.

MIDWIVES ENGAGING WITH MEDIA TO CHANGE DISCOURSE

Dispelling Myths in Media to Undo Harm

The midwives in our study viewed media portrayals of birth as being at best oversimplified and often sensationalist. The depictions of midwifery were often seen as inaccurate and, while midwives reported feeling frustrated about the representation, they were more concerned about the impact that the messages had on women.

> It would just be quite nice to have a TV soap or a film that isn't making birth dramatic and making midwives look like I don't know what! I can't really describe it. It just all seems so dramatic really. (*Participant 8*)

Television programmes in particular were viewed as focusing on the dramatic and midwives felt that the effect was to encourage women to seek more medicalised types of care:

> I think women get frightened when they see things like that. They think, 'Oh my god. If I'm at home and my waters break, I'm in trouble'. Women think it's safer to be in hospital, because that's where all the doctors are, and that kind of thing. (*Participant 1*)

The media's focus on complex and often unusual births was seen as causing fear and 'harm' to women, something that midwives had to subsequently 'undo':

> But I know when ... *One Born Every Minute* had been on the night before, I always felt that I had to undo what *One Born Every Minute* had caused. (*Participant 2*)

These findings reflect the views of midwives in academic literature; for example, in one NHS area a specialist consultant midwife service has been introduced to support fearful women and address concerns about childbirth (Gutteridge 2014). In high-income countries, perinatal and maternal mortality are rare; however, while pregnancy and childbirth has become much safer over the past century, people's perceptions of the associated risk have increased. Thus it could be argued paradoxically that women now fear childbirth more and this anxiety impacts on how they feel they can cope during labour (Eriksson et al. 2005). Otley (2011) determined that there are five main categories of fear that women can experience: "biological (fear of pain); psychological (due to previous traumatic events, personality factors, feelings of helplessness, anxiety about parenthood); social (lack of support, low educational level); cultural (the medicalisation of childbirth, 'horror stories' being passed on); secondary (caused by previous childbirth experiences)" (2011: 215).

The midwives in our study were particularly sensitive to these cultural fears, which they felt were provoked by media representation on reality television, soap operas and in journalistic reporting:

> There's something about people being scared of the unknown. I think it goes back to a deeper social problem that historically women would have seen their sister, mothers giving birth when they were children.... What we did was that we removed birth from people's lives, put it in the hospital, hid it away, so it became not only unseen, but unknown. We've now brought it back into the public arena, but in a sensationalized form. In a way, we've kind of turned back to where we started, but with the sensationalism. (*Participant 9*)

One interviewee singled out the negative portrayal in the media of women (and their partners) who do not want hospital confinement, for example:

...there is less representation of the homebirth scenario or the birth center scenario, and there is a kind of misconception of people being absolutely mad if they would give birth anywhere else other than a hospital. (*Participant 3*)

Another interviewee noted the urge for media to sensationalise:

I have yet to see anything which is not sensationalised. How can that be anything other than alarming?... I think you can see *One Born Every Minute*... I come out of it terrified sometimes! I've only watched it occasionally, but I've sat on the edge of my chair, normally shouting, 'no, don't do that!' That just can't be right. (*Participant 5*)

Discourses of misrepresentation, the dramatic and the unusual abounded. As we have written previously, women are exposed to four different viewpoints on and perceptions of childbirth that include (1) an often stereotypical sensationalised version of the birthing process in media; (2) stories from friends and relatives; (3) antenatal information provided by midwives, doctors and other childbirth educators; and (4) personal experiences of giving birth (Luce et al. 2016). Whilst midwives might be critical of women seeking out programmes that depict inaccurate representations of childbirth, we need to remember that media representations are, for most women, the only opportunity to see a birth. It is these media representations, with which the midwives in our study had problems. Interestingly, when we asked participants about the midwife's responsibility to help change the discourse within the media, a different narrative started to emerge.

Distrust in Talking to the Media

Midwives clearly recognised that they have a responsibility when it comes to the media representation about childbirth. Hundley and colleagues (2015) identified a number of roles for midwives in relation to the media, which ranged from harnessing the power of the media to get positive messages out, to engaging with media producers to ensure better media representation. However, in our study the majority of midwives only felt comfortable in correcting misrepresentations of childbirth in one-to-one conversations with women.

Most of the midwives felt that speaking directly with journalists or media producers was not part of their role. A number of the interviewees indicated a significant distrust of journalists and indicated that they would refuse to do media interviews if asked:

> The less I engage with them the better. I just think they're out for their own ends, whether that's politicians, and maybe you get used to that in your job, but it's [talking to the press] not a pressure that you should have, being a midwife. You should be able to get on and do your job, and not have to deal with all the crap that the media is throwing at you all the time. (*Participant 7*)

> ... it is the fear that what they [midwives] would say potentially would be taken out of context, and also you've got data protection, confidentiality. (*Participant 9*)

In some cases, the distrust of the media was deflected through statements that indicated that the midwife had a professional duty to not speak with the media. This was particularly true with regard to social media as we discuss below.

> We can't bring our employer into disrepute, so it would be risky to speak to a reporter, say, because they might twist what you say and we have to communicate through our communications department, which I think is fair enough.... I think there is just a mistrust of the media because they are not going to understand and they twist it to make it newsworthy. (*Participant 2*)

In *Midwifery Matters* in 2012, Meg Taylor lamented the ways in which midwives were portrayed in the media. She noted that the high standard of care that midwives provide is 'unappreciated by those outside the midwifery field and called for high profile midwives and professional bodies: to make their voices heard in the mass media' (Taylor 2012, pp. 3–6). This sentiment was echoed by many of our interviewees.

> I think that if we don't [engage with media], then we can't really complain if the media puts out the wrong stuff, stuff which is incorrect, sensationalist or well, largely incorrect. Unless we are prepared to stand up to be counted and correct it, I think all midwives, if they read a newspaper and they see something rubbish, they read a magazine and see something

incorrect, they should make a point of writing and sending a correction, because sooner or later editors will get sick of this kind of constant correspondence. That might get them to think, 'do you know what? We'll check our facts before we print'. (*Participant 5*)

While some participants begrudgingly admitted that midwives needed to start engaging with media producers, the general feeling was that professional and regulatory bodies needed to lead by example. We quote one interviewee at length here as it sums up the discussion nicely:

> When you think about some political things that come up, you think, where's the RCM, Royal College of Midwives? I don't see their voice, I see the nurses' voice in that, and I see other professions and I think, where is the midwifery voice? I think that's the problem. We're not loud enough and we're not all the time. We should be there all the time saying, 'this is what we do'. Not just reacting when bad things come out and say this, that, and the other. I think, yes, we should be doing that, and I think what the problem is, I personally think, it might not be other people's perceptions, but we are not political enough as a group. We are a bunch of women doing the job and we're not political. I think we need to be more political. Myself and my colleagues, we're not doing it and people in the practice are not doing it. They're exhausted. They don't have the time to be thinking politically now. They come home from shift and they're just finished. That's the problem. (*Participant 1*)

COMMUNICATING MIDWIFERY IN THE TWENTY-FIRST CENTURY: THE ROLE OF SOCIAL MEDIA

Midwifery, in common with other fields, like higher education, is being subjected to increasing 'consumer' demands and expectation with regard to information. In the twenty-first century that communication and engagement will include the use of social media: 'social media is where the future is, and most importantly, that's where our patients are going to be' (Prasad 2013: 492). Increasingly social media is also the place for professional collaboration and this caused some of the midwives in our study concern.

The midwives in our study understood that women no longer seek out their information about childbirth in books and leaflets, but first turned to the internet. With that comes the knowledge that women are engaging in forums like Mumsnet and that midwives can play a critical role in spreading positive information across the internet.

I have connections with people who have influence [on Twitter], but also I connect with women's groups and midwives groups from an educator's point of view so that I can help educate students and educate people around birth.... I find it a really useful way to keep up to date, but also useful tool to help create perhaps a more positive view around birth. (*Participant 8*)

As we have seen, professional and regulatory bodies have provided guidance and support with engaging with social media. However, Wylie (2014) argues, 'much of the advice given by managers and academics, especially to midwives and student midwives, had been alarmist regarding the risk to an individual's professional registration if they fail to abide by the regulatory framework of the profession' (p. 502). It is clear that some of this fear has passed on to the midwives in this study.

I don't have a Facebook account, and I don't really wish to have a Facebook account. But I feel pressurised to have one, as a lot of interactive things that are to do with midwifery professionally take place there. ... Qualified midwives could lose their jobs if they put up stuff on there, so it's a bit of a battle isn't it? (*Participant 4*)

Others agreed, referring to the NMC Code of practice:

If you start saying unprofessional things, then you could be held up to account for that. You'd have to go in front of the Nursing and Midwifery Council and justify that. ... I'm just worried about my profession. They're forever telling us, 'Be careful what you say online because when it's out there, it's out there'. It's very hard to retract those words. (*Participant 1*)

... some midwives haven't understood the rules around social media and have even lost their registration due to what they have said or done on there. Probably not intentionally meaning to cause any harm, so I think that has potentially frightened midwives from engaging, or making them extra wary or anxious.... there are strict rules and policies on media use when you're a midwife, and you've worked so hard to get your registration so you don't want to lose that. (*Participant 9*)

While overwhelmingly the challenges and 'dangers' of social media concerned the participants, there was only one midwife who did see the benefit of engaging with it.

> I definitely think social media is the most influential medium in terms of childbirth; we live in such a world of social media now, and that can be really influential. You can find a group for everything nowadays, and I think, unfortunately, that's where women go to get their information first. (*Participant 10*)

What became quite clear from listening to the midwives in our study discuss the role of social media in their profession is that they were scared and conflicted when it comes to using social media. Professional and regulatory bodies in several countries including the United Kingdom and Australia have strict guidelines on what can and cannot be posted on social media; and while there is no direct requirement to engage on social media, pregnant women are expecting communication in that sphere. Midwives fear for their jobs if they step out of line and misuse social media. There is a general understanding of what 'stepping out of line' means, yet as Bernadette John (2015) wrote in *World of Irish Nursing & Midwifery*, 'it is essential that we establish where the challenges lie and mitigate for the risks' (47).

Midwives and Media Training

Midwifery is no longer a profession which can afford to ignore the media. Midwives need training in traditional media as well as social media and in how to speak to journalists and stay on topic. Yet, the interviewees in our study were not keen to speak to media without some media training, and some didn't see it as their responsibility at all.

> I'm not doing it [talking to the media] until I've had my media training. I refuse. I'm not speaking until I know what it is. I'm know going to go out there… they take things out of context. I want to know what my parameters are and how you answer questions and don't say things that you don't need to say. (*Participant 1*)

> Well, I would like to talk to the media if I had training on it, but I don't have and I don't feel comfortable. (*Participant 4*)

A more absolute rejection of dealing with the media was expressed by this interviewee:

> If I wanted to go on telly, I would be an actress. I'm not craving that sort of attention. (*Participant 2*)

In an editorial in the *Journal of Clinical Nursing*, Jones and Hayter (2013: 1496) argue just this:
Teaching should be geared towards identifying the strengths and weaknesses of social media, the correct use of privacy settings and the career implications of e-professionalism blunders. It is also important that clinicians involved in mentoring students are engaged with the issues associated with social media and can reinforce good practice from the clinical perspective.

In discussing whether student midwives should have media training, the midwives in our study were split—with half saying student midwives already have too much to think about, while the other half thought there was value in it.

> No, it shouldn't happen above everything else they've got to learn. They have a very full curriculum and more and more stuff gets put in it by policymakers. (*Participant 7*)

> Yeah, to a certain extent [student midwives should have training]. I think so because I think its something that happens quite a lot in the profession. Because things you say could be taken out of context, or could be distorted—like they can take out part of your sentences and make it relate to something else entirely, so I think that's quite difficult." (*Participant 10*)

Tuckett and Turner (2016), in their study on midwifery students' use of social media, found that 97% of Australian students were using Facebook but only 48% of them believed they should not use social media to discuss work matters. The students in this study mainly used social media for social reasons, while only 27% of them thought of social media as a place of educational value. In our study there was some evidence of a difference of opinion between younger and older midwives. In general, older midwives expressed more concern regarding the media, whereas the youngest participant in our study (a 28-year-old, band 5 midwife) thought that media training 'might reduce midwives' fears and anxieties around approaching or being approached by the media'.

While it is clear from our participants that not all midwives necessarily want or will engage with media, it does appear that it would benefit the profession. Midwives need to be more media savvy if they are to counter the negative portrayals of birth and to do this, more training is required. While some interviewees in our study believed curricula were already too busy and full to integrate anything further, this would be the best place to engage new midwives who are entering the profession.

Social media can be harnessed across teaching, and implemented in current assessments; it doesn't have to be onerous, but it does rely on current midwifery educators engaging and learning and using social media themselves.

> I do think we live in this world of social media, and I do think that as a general whole, it's a positive thing. It's much easier to get information now, and it's much easier to access a wide variety of people, geographically as well. You can get in touch with people all across the world and I think that's something that needs to be harnessed, to make positive stories out of it opposed to these negative stories that seem to get so much media attention. (*Participant 10*)

CONCLUSION

This chapter reports findings from a qualitative study that shows midwives and midwifery academics fear engaging with the media. This fear may compound the problem that arises because pregnant women take unrealistic portrayals of birth from both fictional and so-called 'reality' television programmes and digest what they have 'learned' to inform their own pregnancies. While it is clear that a few midwives want to engage with journalists, others definitely do not. The biggest fear is the risk of being misquoted or saying something that should not have been said and the potential for losing a license or bringing an employer into disrepute. Social media presented a significant problem for midwives. They recognised that pregnant women are engaging on social media and perhaps this is an area for providing additional information and care, but with strict regulatory guidelines and a general mistrust of the media, it appears unlikely that the midwifery field as a whole will engage with social media anytime soon.

We feel strongly there is a need for midwives to extend their skillset, and this culture change could first happen on midwifery courses. Student midwives need to be taught how to engage with journalists from all different media, including newspaper, radio, television and online. Education is needed on how to use social media effectively, on how to break through the barriers of Twitter and understand how Facebook can be harnessed to support the work midwives do, while also adhering to regulatory guidelines. For this to occur, however, buy-in is needed from practising midwives, professionals who are willing to learn. They must first engage and then teach those midwives coming behind them.

Midwives have a critical role to play in helping to change media discourse around midwifery and how childbirth and early labour are portrayed in fictional and non-fictional representations. To do that, however, midwives have to be willing to equip themselves with the skills necessary to engage with the media. We are not suggesting that all midwives need to engage with the media, merely to have the knowledge and know-how if ever approached. The midwifery field is changing. Midwives coming into the profession will face more and more demands to use social media and to engage with media to defend their positions. It is our responsibility to make sure that every midwife entering our profession is equipped to tackle whatever challenge is thrown her way, even if that is dealing with challenging media professionals.

Editor's Note: In this chapter, the editors argued that midwives need to engage with media. In the next chapter, Prof. Hannah Dahlen, National Media Spokesperson for the Australian College of Midwives, delves deeper into how midwives can work with the media and outlines a strategy for dealing with all forms of media.

REFERENCES

Clement, S. 1997. Childbirth on television. *British Journal of Midwifery* 5 (1): 37–42.
Dahlen, H.G., and S. Caplice. 2014. What do midwives fear? *Women and Birth* 27: 266–270.
Declercq, E.R., et al. 2006. *Listening to mothers II: Report of the second national US survey of women's childbearing experiences*. New York: Childbirth Connection.
Department of Health. 1970. *The peel report*. London: HMSO.
Donnison, J. 1977. *Midwives and medical men*. London: Heineman.
Eriksson, C., G. Westman, and K. Hamberg. 2005. Experiential factors associated with childbirth related fear in Swedish women and men: A population based study. *Journal of Psychosomatic Obstetrics and Gynecology* 26 (1): 63–72.
Gutteridge, K. 2014. Q&A interview: Katherine Gutteridge. *MIDIRS*. http://www.midirs.org/qa-interview-kathryn-gutteridge/.
Hundley, V., E. Duff, J. Dewberry, A. Luce, and E. van Teijlingen. 2014. Fear in childbirth: Are the media responsible? *MIDIRS Midwifery Digest* 24 (4): 444–447.
Hundley, V., E. van Teijlingen, and A. Luce. 2015. Do midwives need to be more media savvy? *MIDIRS Midwifery Digest* 25 (1): 5–10.

John, B. 2015. Online professionalism. *World of Irish Nursing and Midwifery* 23 (7): 47.
Jones, C., and M. Hayter. 2013. Editorial: Social media use by nurses and midwives: A 'recipe for disaster' or a 'force for good'? *Journal of Clinical Nursing* 22: 1495–1496.
Laja, S. 2011. Trusts reveal staff abuse of social media. *Guardian.* https://www.theguardian.com/healthcare-network/2011/nov/09/trusts-reveal-staff-abuse-of-social-media-facebook.
Luce, A., M. Cash, M. Hundley, H. Cheyne, E. van Teijlingen, and C. Angell. 2016. Is it realistic? The portrayal of pregnancy and childbirth in the media. *BMC Pregnancy and Childbirth.* Accessible Online: https://bmcpregnancychildbirth.biomedcentral.com/articles/10.1186/s12884-016-0827-x.
Maclean, E. 2014. What to expect when you're expecting? Representations of birth in British newspapers. *British Journal of Midwifery* 22: 8. Published online: http://www.magonlinelibrary.com/doi/abs/10.12968/bjom.2014.22.8.580.
Nursing and Midwifery Council. 2016. *Guidance on using social media responsibily.* London: NMC. https://www.nmc.org.uk/globalassets/sitedocuments/nmc-publications/social-media-guidance.pdf.
Otley, H. 2011. Fear of childbirth: Understanding the causes, impact and treatment. *British Journal of Midwifery* 19 (4): 215–220.
Prasad, B. 2013. Social media, health care and social networking. *Gastrointestinal Endoscopy* 77 (3): 492–495.
RCM. 2014. *Social networking—Dos and don'ts.* London: RCM i-learn.
Riddoch. L., and L. Orr (n.d.) *Handle with care: A guide to responsible media reporting of violence against women.* Zero Tolerance. http://www.endviolenceagainstwomen.org.uk/data/files/ZT_Handle_With_Care_Media_Guide.pdf.
Schwitzer, G., G. Mudur, D. Henry, A. Wilson, M. Goozner, et al. 2005. What are the roles and responsibilities of the media in disseminating health information? *PLOS Medicine* 2 (7): e215. doi:10.1371/journal.pmed.0020215. http://journals.plos.org/plosmedicine/article?id=10.1371/journal.pmed.0020215.
Taylor, M. 2012. Midwives in the media. *Midwifery Matters* 132: 3–6.
Tuckett, A., and C. Turner. 2016. Do you use social media? A student into new nursing and midwifery graduates uptake of social media. *International Journal of Nursing Practice* 22: 197–204.
WHO and IASP. 2008/2017. *Preventing suicide: A resource for media professionals.* Geneva: WHO. http://www.who.int/mental_health/prevention/suicide/resource_media.pdf.
Wylie, L. 2014. The social media revolution. *British Journal of Midwifery* 22 (7): 502–506.

CHAPTER 8

Working With the Media: The Power, the Pitfalls and the Possibilities

Hannah G. Dahlen

Abstract Hannah G. Dahlen has been working with the media as spokesperson for the Australian College of Midwives for 20 years now and has undertaken research into media representations of midwives and obstetricians. There is enormous potential power when midwives work effectively with the media. Having a public voice enables you to shift thinking about childbirth and can be a part of shifting paradigms of understanding around the profession of midwifery. The political power of a positive midwifery presence in the media cannot be underestimated. However, working with the media also takes persistence, patience, resilience and an understanding about how messages are best delivered to be effective. There are significant pitfalls; and the media can turn quickly and demonise midwives. In the world of every-expanding social media, effective messages can be delivered quickly and effectively but cyber bullying is ever present and can be very distressing to deal with. The higher profile midwives become in the media the more they are exposed to this. This chapter will focus on tips for midwives in learning to deal with the media and present themselves in the best possible light. It will explore

H.G. Dahlen (✉)
School of Nursing and Midwifery, Western Sydney University,
Sydney, Australia
e-mail: h.dahlen@westernsydney.edu.au

© The Author(s) 2017
A. Luce et al. (eds.), *Midwifery, Childbirth and the Media*,
DOI 10.1007/978-3-319-63513-2_8

the pitfalls and help midwives identify skills that can help them maximise their message and realise the possibilities. It will also reflect on research undertaken into the representations of midwives and obstetricians in the media and how negative stereotypes can be altered.

Keywords Media · Blogs · Internet · Dealing with media · Midwives

Introduction

I have been working with the media as spokesperson for the Australian College of Midwives for nearly 20 years now and have undertaken research into media representations of midwives and obstetricians and what women say in blogs and in internet discussion forums. There is enormous potential power in working effectively with the media. Having a public voice enables you to shift thinking about childbirth; and you in turn can be a part of shifting paradigms of understanding around women's issues and the profession of midwifery. The political power of a positive midwifery presence in the media cannot be underestimated. However, working with the media also takes persistence, patience, resilience and an understanding about how messages are best delivered to be effective. There are significant pitfalls; and the media can quickly turn on, and demonise, midwives. In the world of ever-expanding social media, strong messages can be delivered quickly and effectively but cyber-bullying and trolling is ever-present and this can be very distressing for midwives to deal with. The higher midwives' profiles become in the media the more they are exposed to this.

This chapter will explore how the media works from my 20 years of working with it as a midwife and why the media may represent birth and midwives in the way it does. The term *media* will be used to refer to print, radio, television, film and the web. Social media will also be discussed briefly: Twitter, Facebook, Instagram, among others. This chapter will provide helpful tips for midwives in learning to deal with the media and present themselves in the best possible light. It will also explore the common pitfalls midwives may inadvertently experience when engaging with the media and help midwives identify skills that can help them maximise their message and realise the possibilities. It will also reflect on research undertaken into the representations of midwives and obstetricians in the media and what women's voices in blogs and internet discussion forums can tell us.

The First Lesson Is Patience and the Final Lesson Is Resilience

When we work with the media we find our voice. When we find our voice, we get others to listen. When others listen, we can change thinking. When thinking is changed, then in time the world can be changed as well. When midwives work successfully with the media they can channel their passion in an immensely powerful way and be a part of shifting paradigms of understanding around the midwifery profession, and this can ultimately lead to changes in the way the profession of midwifery is seen in the world and the kind of care made available to women. The political power of a good midwifery presence in the media cannot be underestimated and I have spent much of my career working to make this happen. Whether it is providing the public with information on continuity of midwifery care models or making complex research accessible to consumers, the media is a great avenue for informing and exposing women to choice and options of care. Patience is critical and it is the first lesson you need to learn, as you cannot expect things to change with one media opportunity and you are only one cog in the wheel of change that turns ever so slowly. As I have written before, 'I have learned that you say it once in the media and no one gets it; you say it twice and they spell your name correctly, if you are lucky; you say it ten times and they ask better questions; you say it a hundred times and they start to use your words in an intelligent way showing they understand what you said; you say it a thousand times and they no longer ask you as by now it is seen as self evident' (Dahlen 2015).

There are many other skills needed after you have conquered patience, such as persistence, reliability, a good sense of humour and a giant dose of humility (Dahlen 2015). Once I turned up on the set of a well-known Sydney morning TV show at the crack of dawn for an interview on the rising caesarean section rate, only to be told the section had just been cancelled due to a breaking news story. I was very gracious about it and said I understood completely. I drove home and got back in bed with a cup of tea, only to switch on the TV and discover the breaking news story was that Whitney Houston had admitted to taking drugs. At the time I laughed but sadly a few years later this did become a major news story with her overdose widely reported. Later that morning a large bunch of flowers was sent to me from the TV station thanking me for my good humour about the entire event. They asked me back many times more after this. Never burn your bridges no matter how much you are screaming inside. You may think what you have to say is the most important thing in the world, but that is not necessary what mainstream media thinks. Bide your time and remain available and calm and they will want you again. While they call you 'the talent' in media when you are asked for comment, don't get deluded that they actually think you are talented! Humility is needed in this job, as Whitney Houston will win hands down against a story about midwives or birth.

Resilience is another attribute you need when working with the media. I have watched potential media talent curl up and die and never try again when they experience their first hostile interview, or are subjected to cyber-trolling, or when they get completely misquoted, or forget the microphone was still on and say something unfortunate that gets used. A big mistake I made early on in my experience with the media was in the year 2000 when women were booking caesarean sections/inductions, or delaying birth, in order to have their baby born in the last or next century. I said to the journalist it was a moral issue at some point in the interview and the headline was *Y2K Kids Immoral*. I learned never to use strong or easily manipulated language after that. Learning from these incidents or mistakes just makes you better and wiser, but they can be very distressing. Having to do radio interviews the next day after the *Y2K Kids Immoral* article and explain that I did not mean what was now plastered all over the front page of the paper was painful. I have experienced several cyber attacks from well-known cyber trolls and I have learned not to respond, not to react, to take a deep breath and finally remember it is about them not you. Even better, don't read the comments and don't respond to abuse as is just fuels the issue and drains your energy. I discuss this more later in this chapter. It is friends and family that get you through, reminding you why you do what you do and that it is not about you anyway.

THE MEDIA THRIVES ON DRAMA BECAUSE WE DO AS HUMANS

There are so many examples of how the media thrives on drama that I could fill this entire book with them, but here is one example. In 2009 the lovely and much respected Dr. Denis Walsh, an Australian born but United Kingdom residing midwife gave a paper on normal birth, which is his area of interest and research. He was unaware a journalist was sitting in the audience. Shortly after this *The Telegraph* ran the story 'Women "should go through pain" in childbirth, says male midwife' (Gardham 2009). The headline and the article were crafted to inflame:

> The pain involved in childbirth serves a purpose and more women should go through it in order to prepare themselves for the responsibility of bringing up a baby, according to Dr Denis Walsh. Dr Walsh, a senior midwife and associate professor in midwifery at Nottingham University, said, 'A large number of women want to avoid pain. Some just don't fancy the pain [of childbirth]. More women should be prepared to withstand pain'.

The fact Denis was a man added to the drama and it played out across the world. In Australia I had around 20 media interviews in one day and by the end of the day people had lost track of what the story was about and were making sharp instruments to insert in Denis's orifices. In reality most people did little more than read the headline of the story and react. I tried to bring a moderate approach to the debate in Australia saying there was a time and a place for epidurals, especially when labour was long and hard. In the end there was nothing much to do but wait for the drama to simmer down and become yesterday's news. If Denis had not been a man I think perhaps it would have been less controversial. Later when I chatted to Denis about the issue he told me his two sisters in Australia had interesting reactions. One put on lipstick and waited for the media to arrive and the other wanted to change her name! And so sums up the varied response we have as humans to drama!

The reality is that many in the media love drama simply because we, the consumers of this media, love drama - as long as it is happening to someone else and not us. Drama, very simply, entertains. Humans love a good drama and journalists are humans and also know this about their audience. What we don't realise is drama also frightens over time. There continues to be debate about the impact for example of reality television programs (e.g., *One Born Every Minute*) that portray birth as dramatic and risky and whether this has an impact on decisions made by women and fear of birth in society (Kennedy et al. 2009; Bick 2010; Luce et al. 2016). These TV shows may also perpetuate the medicalisation of childbirth by the absence of normal birth portrayals (Luce et al. 2016).

While midwives often criticise the media for its obsession with drama when it comes to birth, and the way it focuses on bad stories instead of good ones, we have to accept a certain amount of responsibility for this as we also use bad news stories (e.g., caesarean section morbidity) to put across our points in support of normal birth. The media plays a strong role in marketing fear through how it represents childbirth and the health professionals involved (Gardner 2008; Dahlen 2010, 2011a). The problem is that media depictions are partial truths and can create a false reality, which in turn can become the established truth (Dahlen 2015).

Media theories range from describing audiences as passive, to arguing that audiences are active and construct their own meanings from the media they consume (Seale 2003). In between these two positions lies the bulk of media consumption theory. Seale (2003), who is a leader in this area says audiences seek emotional stimulation through dramatised contrasts that have an entertaining effect. Fear and anxiety, for example, may be aroused so that they are experienced as a contrast to security and pleasure (Seale 2003). It is hardly surprising then that childbirth becomes a focus for media attention.

Media health stories often oppose life with the threat, or reality of death. In doing this fundamental anxiety that we face as humans is explored. Doctors are often the focus, or central characters in TV medical dramas because they are seen as making life and death decisions (Seale 2003); they are also often male. Another common media technique that is used to generate dramatic effect is by taking opposites and putting them side-by-side. Death during a homebirth is a prime example. What should have been life and a new beginning becomes death and ending. The anger generated then gets targeted at the so-called selfish parents (particularly the woman), who are seen to have chosen their own selfish needs and comfort over the safety of the innocent baby. This raises the good and bad mother constructs, leading to misunderstanding and blame. You see the same issue in polarised views on vaccination.

The media also likes to use what are called 'twitchers', and this involves using news items that disrupt expectations in order to stimulate emotions. An example of this would be a baby found in a rubbish tip or born on the side of the road. These images contrast strongly with what we expect should happen, which is that birth for the majority of the developed world occurs in medically clean environments. Both the media and society also have 'templates' about what is considered normal or acceptable and when these 'templates' are reversed or changed they can achieve a dramatic or entertaining effect (Seale 2003). Seale (2003) describes a meta-narrative threaded through media reports containing five key elements that constitute a series of core oppositions (Table 8.1).

Table 8.1 Five key elements constitute a series of core oppositions

1. The dangers of modern life-fear and safety (birth, death, damage)
2. Villains and freaks (too posh to push, lay midwives, bad mothers)
3. Victimhood (innocent baby/mother)
4. Professional heroes (midwives and doctors)
5. Lay heroes (taxi-driver delivers baby)

Seale (2003)

WHY BAD IS STRONGER THAN GOOD WHEN IT COMES TO THE MEDIA?

The language of risk and fear and death predominates in media reports because these issues are of importance to humans. Understanding the psychology of fear helps us to understand why the media functions the way it does and what strategies are needed to overcome fear. Fear serves to protect us and Darwinians believe that in fact the early humans who were most afraid were most likely to survive (Dahlen 2010). Baumeister et al. (2001) showed the greater power that 'bad events' have over 'good events' is found in everyday events, major life events (e.g., trauma), close relationship outcomes, social network patterns, interpersonal interactions and learning processes. Bad emotions, bad parents and bad feedback have more impact than good ones, and bad information is processed more thoroughly than good (Baumeister et al. 2001). The self is more motivated to avoid bad self-definitions than to pursue good ones (Baumeister et al. 2001). Bad impressions and bad stereotypes are quicker to form and more resistant to disconfirmation than good ones (Baumeister et al. 2001). In fact, Baumeister et al. (2001) found that there were hardly any exceptions to this rule. Taken together they concluded that these findings suggest that 'bad is stronger than good', as a general principle across a broad range of psychological phenomena. This helps us to understand why drama and death is more often reported and of interest to the media than a problem free birth. However, it is not all doom and gloom, as Baumeister and colleagues point out that 'many events can overcome the psychological effects of a single bad one. When equal measures of good and bad are present, however the psychological effects of bad ones outweigh those of the good one'. So it is an uphill battle, but it is not an impossible one. Murphy-Lawless (1998, p. 229) says, 'If I were to extract only two words whereby to classify the concerns of contemporary obstetric practice, they would include not birth, but risk and death'. I would argue this is not just the concern of obstetrics, as humans this concern is hardwired into us. It should not surprise us then when the media prioritises this paradigm and midwives have to work so hard to have the positive messages about birth and women's capacity heard above fear and the messages about women and birth as catastrophe.

Pregnancy, Birth and Parenting Are No Longer Women's Secret Business

Midwives no longer have the option of not becoming media savvy and getting politically engaged if they want to maintain/enhance their profession and improve options and outcomes for women, babies and families. Pregnancy, birth and parenting are no longer women's secret business; they are in the public domain. Childbirth documentaries such as *One Born Every Minute* hold people captive in their lounge rooms at night, while high-ranking shows like *Call the Midwife* spark the imagination of the world and transcend cultures. Birth websites and blogs abound and women can post photos on Instagram of their pregnancies on a daily basis (sometimes multiple times a day).

Universities and Academics Are Learning To Engage With the Media

Researchers and universities have learned to get active in the media, putting out media releases when new studies come out, writing complex findings in language accessible to a layperson in mediums such as *The Conversation*. Translation of research findings into practice has become not only the catchcry of the modern university but academics are now assessed and promoted according to their ability to translate their research into practice. Midwifery is not immune from this, as in many countries midwifery is now taught in universities and midwives are increasingly becoming highly influential researchers. In many ways we have the enormous advantage of dealing with mothers and babies, both are highly valued and provide photographic opportunities that the media love.

Researchers increasingly develop good relationships with journalists and become accessed as experts on matters they become renowned for. I, for example, edit material and appear in video content on several parenting websites in Australia, such as *Raising Children Network*, *Baby Centre*, and others. For years I wrote for *Australian Parents* magazine. This gives midwives the opportunity to make sure the content is evidence based and provides women with options of care.

SOUNDS GREAT, BUT...

I have engaged, and do engage with all forms of media (TV, film radio, newspapers, magazines, websites, The Conversation, blogs) and social media (Facebook, Twitter, Instagram), and mostly this has worked well; but there are definite downsides and big mistakes can be made. The first downside is that engaging with the media/social media can become obsessive and exhausting. When you wake up in the morning and the first thing you do is check your social media feed it is a sign it is starting to rule rather than assist your life. The more you communicate, the more others communicate with you, so if you think being efficient in your responses is being efficient you will actually find you are just creating more and more work for yourself.

Every time you get a win in the media with a positive normal birth and/or midwifery story you will inevitably generate a backlash. Where I live in New South Wales (NSW), just this month, we had two conflicting articles in one week: first an article advocating the benefits of continuity of midwifery care due the positive consumer response during a NSW State wide satisfaction survey. A couple of days later another article in the same paper by the same journalist slammed midwives as the advocates of a normal birth ideology that was damaging mothers and babies. There is little doubt in my mind that the positive story had led to objections from some of our very vocal and anti midwife obstetricians and the journalist had felt the need to balance the state of play so to speak. This backlash will not just come from the media, who love to entertain with drama, and nothing fits this better than midwives and obstetricians going at it hammer and tongs, but it will also come from those who feel their agenda and power threatened. A normal birth story celebrating the benefits of normal birth will bring out the birth trauma groups and right-wing journalists along with some obstetricians. Equally an article on normal birth being associated with damage of women and babies will bring out the natural birth groups, left wing journalists and midwives. It can feel like an exhausting never ending back and forth which sadly only increases women's fear and distrust in health professionals and in their own capacity to give birth.

Cyber trolls will become a reality in your life if you become successful in your media and social media presence. Dr. Amy, otherwise known as the Skeptical OB, is particularly venomous and gathers in her wake damaged women and angry obstetricians. Some of her classic quotes about me are cutting and you have to develop a thick skin. She has used the following headings for her blogs over the years (and there is much, much more):

> Hannah Dahlen has never met a dead baby she couldn't exploit for her own purpose.
>
> Are Hannah Dahlen and Australian midwives trying to trick people, or just ignorant?
>
> Hannah Dahlen, perhaps you can explain how a mother bonds with a dead baby?
>
> Hannah Dahlen tries to lie with statistics...again. (The Skeptical OB)

Don't get offended and hurt—expect it. I often comfort my colleagues who are under attack and urge them to wear it as a badge of honour. If you are not being noticed, you are not saying anything and no one is listening. The more successful you are in the media and in social media the harsher the attacks from cyber trolls. The most important lesson you need to learn now is never stoop to their level. I always ignore them and treat them as you would a naughty dog by turning your back on them. At other times I leave it to others to respond, but I never descend to their level. Making it personal means you have already lost the argument.

DEPICTIONS OF MIDWIVES AND OBSTETRICIANS IN THE MEDIA

The media both creates and reflects public opinion and the way midwives and obstetricians are depicted in the media (Dahlen 2015). I published a study into one year's worth of web-based news reports from around the world on midwives and obstetricians in 2012 (Dahlen and Homer 2012). In total I analysed 522 web-based news reports mentioning the words *midwives*, *midwife* and *midwifery* and 564 mentioning the words *obstetricians* and *obstetrics*. You can read the full paper in *Birth* (Dahlen and Homer 2012). In this study I found obstetricians were more likely to be reported and consulted as 'experts' on pregnancy and birth and they enjoyed greater public recognition compared to midwives. Midwives were more likely to be depicted as struggling to be a mainstream option of maternity care and they were affected in this struggle by lack of funding, insurance, workforce issues and numerous legislative barriers. The conclusion of this paper was that while midwives have increasing public acceptance they still struggle with recognition, whereas obstetricians are clearly recognised for what they do and are seen as an authority in the area of childbirth. This lack of recognition was more evident in countries where midwifery was not a mainstream option, such as the United States. The number of web-based news reports on midwives and obstetricians also reflected the prominence of the professions in the respective countries. There were many more reports about midwives for example in the United Kingdom compared to obstetricians, and this was the complete reverse in the United States, where midwifery is still not a mainstream option. As the media both reflects and creates opinion, working strategically with the media gives midwives the opportunity to more accurately reflect and to create new norms in society. It was apparent that the highest number of mentions of midwives and most positive mentions of midwives occurred in the month of May when International Day of the Midwife occurs. This is the opportunity for an annual strategy where midwives can promote their profession in a positive way.

This recognition given to obstetrics allows the biomedical voice to remain dominant in public discourse. Jordan (1997) said the power of authoritative knowledge is not that it is correct but that it counts. The fact that obstetricians are consulted in the media as experts in pregnancy and birth, more than midwives, shapes the public's view of which profession has the most authority and expertise when it comes to childbirth. The discourse of medicine is very different to that of midwifery with a disease focus and language of risk and a much greater emphasis on the importance of technology to make birth safe. The language used in the media reports illustrated a dichotomy between the two professions that is real but then becomes reinforced. This subtle but powerful portrayal of the professions cannot help but have an impact on the way the birth is seen by the general public and how relevant midwives are perceived to be.

This is a clear message to our profession that we have to find ways to increase public recognition of our expertise and reframe midwifery as a highly relevant profession for childbearing women (Dahlen and Homer 2012). The media can be an effective way to do this but it can equally backfire on midwives too as it can both sanctify and crucify the profession and it has the ability to instil fear into consumers regarding certain birth choices and health professionals (Dahlen 2009, 2010). One of the main reasons this happens is the media's love of the dramatic, as we have already discussed.

Making Sense Our of Blogs and Internet Discussion Forums

Lessons From Vaginal Birth After Caesarean Section Blogs

I led a study into what women wrote in blogs about vaginal birth after caesarean section (VBAC) (Dahlen and Homer 2011). We analysed 311 internet discussions over a one-year period (November 2007 to October 2008). Most of these blogs originated from the United States. We found, interestingly, that more blogs were written during the Northern Hemisphere winter months than during other seasons, showing that when it is cold and people are indoors more they seem to interact more with social media and the internet. The main theme identified was a dichotomy in philosophical framework women held about birth. We described this as a 'motherbirth' or 'childbirth' framework (Dahlen and Homer 2011). Whether women eventually blogged that they chose a VBAC or repeat caesarean, or the extent to which they pursued their birth choice depended on whether they came from a perspective that a 'good parent sacrifices themselves for their baby (prioritises the baby) and takes no risks' (childbirth) or that 'giving birth matters to the woman and a happy, healthy mother is a happy healthy baby (mother and baby have equal priority)' (motherbirth) (Dahlen and Homer 2011). Several themes were identified, including 'surviving the damage', 'inadequate bodies', 'choice and control', 'fearing and trusting birth', 'negotiating the system' and 'minimising or overestimating risk'. This study enabled us to understand more about the positions society, and hence also women, take on what makes a good mother when it comes to birth choices such as VBAC and how women embody that positioning.

Lessons from Internet Discussion Forums on Miscarriage

Another study led by Debra Betts, one of my PhD students from Western Sydney University, examined women's experiences of threatened miscarriage through examining postings to Internet discussion forums (Betts et al. 2013). Betts collected Google alerts for subjects mentioning miscarriage over a seven-month period (April to November 2011) and analysed these discussion forums using thematic analysis. The study found that one of the overarching themes was one of 'a search for hope and understanding'. The study found that internet discussion forums were used by women to seek hope and support they felt they were not receiving from their healthcare professionals. Women urged each other to remain hopeful despite a negative medical prognosis. A reason for hope was typically given within the postings through women sharing their experiences of how they continued with a healthy pregnancy, often after being told that they had miscarried or would miscarry. These were discussed as triumphs in the face of medical advice that there was no hope; and the postings clearly challenged medical expertise:

> I had bleeding at 5, 8 and 10 weeks of varying levels. Each time I was told a miscarriage was inevitable and in one case was told to go to the hospital to get some medication to finish the miscarriage off. Well good thing I didn't as my 'miscarriage' is now 2!(HM/92/3). (cited in Betts et al. 2013, p. 652)

There was an acceptance of a lay expertise within the forums that was valid enough to challenge medical expertise, though at times some of the advice given was clearly problematic (Betts et al. 2013).

> Really?? He said it could be a complete miscarriage?? That's ridiculous because a small amount of bleeding as you've described with I'm assuming not much pain if any? That's all normal!! You know what honey the more I think about it, the more I believe you're fine!! Honestly if you were in a lot more pain with a lot more blood then yeah I'd say be worried but seriously these docs should know what normal pregnancy symptoms are(LA/86/2). (cited in Betts et al. 2013, p. 653)

This sort of research enables us as health professionals to not only understand where women go to get their information but how we can perhaps better frame our care so what we say and the way we say it can be more acceptable to women. However, it also alerts us to the power of peer support and the need to harness this more in health and not try to be everything to all people.

Tips for Dealing With the Media

Below are some practical tips for dealing with different kinds of media:

Media releases

- Write short, clear sentences and a short paragraph for each concept.
- Provide a clever headline, as it might be used in news reports.
- Provide strong defining quotes journalists can use and attribute the quote to someone who can be contacted for interview.
- Provide access to a woman with a new baby who has agreed to be interviewed and photographed (journalists will often ask for mother and baby pictures). The less work a journalist has to do, the more likely the story will run.
- Deliver the media release to a key journalist you trust the day before you wish your announcement to be released. Give this journalist 'the scoop'. Once the story is in the media, then make your announcement.
- Media releases cost money so put them out when you have something important to say and don't make them longer than one page.
- If you want immediate impact send out your media release Monday–Wednesday. Audiences are smaller at the weekend, so aim for earlier in the week announcements.
- Be prepared for your story to be pushed farther down the news agenda if breaking news occurs. You have no control over this.

Newspapers

- Know that anything you say is 'on the record' and can be used. If you do not want them to use something, then tell them it is 'off the record' BEFORE you say it, or just don't say it at all.
- If you are responding to a news request for comment, take your time. You can always ask for an hour to get a response to them so you have time to prepare.
- If a journalist is happy with an e-mailed response to a question, then put your words in quotation marks and it will be printed verbatim.

- Know that journalists have to provide both sides of the story, so they will interview an obstetrician for another point of view. Anticipate what will be said and explain the deficit in the argument.
- You do not always have to respond to an interview request. Sometimes saying nothing is the wisest option. Sometimes this makes the story go away.
- All you need is one good newspaper story and all the other media will follow: radio, TV, magazines, internet sites and blogs.
- Pages 1 and 3 are the best exposure, but you will have no control over this (more than likely, neither will the journalist!).
- Always ask if the story will appear online and will it be on the homepage. This is where maximum exposure takes place, even if it is just a link.

Radio

- Live radio is best as editing is limited.
- Live radio is also risky; you need to know your stuff and if you say something you didn't mean to, there's no going back!
- Pre-recorded radio news segments need to be short and to the point. Write down what you are going to say.
- Sound warm and engaging as all people have is your voice to go by.

Television and film

- You have little time to speak. Make sure you have short sound-bites about the key points you want to get across (3–5 seconds, or one short sentence).
- You need to look professional and sound professional.
- You need to be friendly and confident. People may not remember what you say, but your presence will convey an important message.
- Never wear checks, spots or green. Remember they usually film you from waist up so concentrate your attentions there.
- Be really nice to the cameraperson as they are in control of how they frame you in the shot.
- Always check your background and don't let a cameraperson position you squinting into the sun—you will look cranky and old!

- Put some makeup on, especially around your eyes as people are drawn to eyes.
- Always assume that your mic is live and you are being recorded, even after the interview is over.
- You will be called 'the talent' in TV but don't let it go to your head it does not mean they think you are talented.

Parenting magazines and websites

- Follow the same guidelines for newspapers.
- You generally can organise the time for this and they will tell you the questions they want to ask. It's very relaxed.

Writing for *The Conversation* as an academic midwife

- Pitch your idea to a health editor.
- Write like you would explain your research at dinner party full of non-health workers.
- Be willing to have your piece rewritten.
- Be prepared to deal with all kinds of comments that may eventuate.

Previously published in (Dahlen 2015).

What you need to *know* when working with the media
- Know what you say is what you believe.
- Know what you say can be verified.
- Know what you say may not be what is printed.
- Know how to keep calm and polite regardless of what questions you face.
- Know how to breathe otherwise you sound breathless and unsure.
- Know how to let go and laugh about it.
- Know how to be humble.
- Know that you don't really know that much and be okay with it.

Previously published in (Dahlen 2015).

Conclusion

Midwives need to understand how the media works and why it tends to work the way it does; otherwise they could easily get depressed and feel completely defeated by the negativity and the daily battle. I hope you have found the tips for dealing with the media and the way you can use media for research useful. For me it all felt worth it when in November 2012 I was named in the *Sydney Morning Herald*'s list of 100 'people who change our city for the better'. I was nominated in the category of leading 'science and knowledge thinkers'. I am told a journalist nominated me. It felt like all those early morning calls, hideous make-up sessions and late nights of worry finally paid off. Remember to be patient and resilient and that 'successfully working with the media is like being a lighthouse. No matter the weather, you must be strong, reliable and able to outlast any storm' (Dahlen 2015).

Editor's Note: In this chapter Dahlen outlined her own experience of working with the media, using it to provide advice and tools for midwives to use when engaging with the media. She argued that midwives need to understand how the media works and why it works the way it does. In our next chapter, Sheena and Anna Byrom explore the world of social media and explain how midwives can use social media to harness information dissemination.

References

Baumeister, R., E. Bratslavsky, C. Finenauer, and K. Vohs. 2001. Bad is stronger than good. *Review of General Psychology* 5: 323–370.

Betts, D., H.G. Dahlen, and C.A. Smith. 2013. A search for hope and understanding: An analysis of threatened miscarriage internet forums. *Midwifery* (in press). Accepted manuscript 26th December 2013.

Bick, D. 2010. Media portrayal of birth and the consequences of misinformation. *Midwifery* 26: 147–148.

Dahlen, H. 2009. Homebirths or births at home: It simply is not the same thing. *ABC Unleashed*. http://www.abc.net.au/unleashed/stories/s2543589.htm.

Dahlen, H. 2010. Undone by fear? Deluded by trust? *Midwifery* 26: 156–162.

Dahlen, H. 2011a. Perspectives on risk or risk in perspective? *Essentially MIDIRS* 2: 17–21.

Dahlen, H. 2011b. Celebrity pregnancy myth busters. *Health and Wellbeing*, Downloaded January 9th 2013. http://health.ninemsn.com.au/pregnancy/labourandbirth/695075/celebrity-pregnancy-myth-busters.

Dahlen, H.G. 2015. Working with the media: The good, the bad and the funny. *Essentially MIDIRS* 6: 14–18.
Dahlen, H., and C. Homer 2011. Motherbirth or childbirth? A prospective analysis of vaginal birth after caesarean blogs. *Midwifery*, 29 (2): 167–173.
Dahlen, H.G., and C.S. Homer 2012. Web-based news reports on midwives compared with obstetricians: A prospective analysis. *Birth* 39 (1): 48–56. doi:10.1111/j.1523-536X.2011.00512.x. Epub 2012 Jan 9.
Gardham, D. 2009. Women 'should go through pain' in childbirth, says male midwife. *The Telegraph*, July 12.
Gardner, D. 2008. *Risk: The science and politics of fear*. London: Virgin Books.
Jordan, B. 1997. Authoritative knowledge and its construction. In *Childbirth and authoritative knowledge: Cross-cutural perspectives*, eds. R. Davis-Floyd, and C. Sargent, 55–79. Berkeley: University of California Press.
Kennedy, H.P., K. Nardini, R. Mcleod-Waldo, and L. Ennis. 2009. Top-selling childbirth advice books: A discourse analysis. *Birth* 36: 318–324.
Luce, A., M. Cash, V. Hundley, H. Cheyne, E. Van Teijlingen, and C. Angell. 2016. "Is it realistic?" The portrayal of pregnancy and childbirth in the media. *BMC Pregnancy and Childbirth* 16. doi:10.1186/s12884-016-0827-x.
Murphy-Lawless, J. 1998. *Reading birth and death: A history of obstetric thinking*. Bloomington: Indiana University Press.
Seale, C. 2003. Health and media: An overview. *Sociology of Health and Illness* 25: 513–531.

CHAPTER 9

Around the World in 80 Tweets—Social Media and Midwifery

Sheena Byrom and Anna Byrom

Abstract In this chapter social media will be presented and reviewed by exploring its impact on midwifery and maternity services, considering global perspectives. It will begin by positioning the opportunities social media presents to midwives, maternity care workers, in addition to childbearing women and their families. A summary of the range of social media platforms available will be presented, and will include an analysis of the increasing utilisation of social media as an important aspect of health promotion and health care. The ongoing maturation of social media technology has broadened the scope for individuals to be heard, and to voice their opinions. This has huge implications for those using and providing maternity care, as service users can share their feedback on the care they've received to the whole world, at the touch of the button. Online blogging is competing with written academic articles for disseminating research and opinion, and the use of social media in increasing readership

S. Byrom (✉)
University of Central Lancashire, Preston, England, UK
e-mail: sheenabyrom@mac.com

A. Byrom
Royal College of Midwives, Marylebone, England, UK
e-mail: abyrom@uclan.ac.uk

© The Author(s) 2017
A. Luce et al. (eds.), *Midwifery, Childbirth and the Media*,
DOI 10.1007/978-3-319-63513-2_9

of high-quality papers through making them more accessible. Social media offers opportunities to maternity workers to access influential leaders and experts, as there are no hierarchies in cyberspace. This in itself presents unlimited opportunities for all parties, and maximises potential for increased social capital through community engagement. It also increases visibility, the chance for student and newly qualified midwives to test out ideas, and then to gain support for taking them forwards. But there needs to be caution, and some health care professionals lack knowledge of the importance of professional integrity and the power or demise of their digital footprint. The chapter will offer a practical guide for midwives on how best to access, utilise and maximise social media avenues for learning from conference and events, networking, lobbying for change, professional development, research, relationship building, communication and midwifery promotion. It will include examples of how social media has acted as a change agent in health care arenas, where the digital space has offered a platform for innovation and engagement, enabling radical change through building supportive networks. The chapter will explore the importance of modelling positive behaviours online, how to stay safe, and to remain within professional boundaries for both personal and professional cyber identities. Social media is here to stay, and the overall focus of this chapter will be about how to use it well.

Keywords Twitter · Tweets · Social media · Midwives · Guidance

Introduction—The Global Picture

We are evolving, and the social media era is well and truly here to stay. The world is becoming smaller due to advances in transportation, television and internet access, with digital technology developments and usage rapidly exploding since the late 1990s. The use of social media has tripled since 2007 (Ofcom 2015), with a reported 2.3 billion active social media users as of January 2016, representing a 10% growth since 2015 and demonstrating a 31% penetration of the total global population (We Are Social 2016). However, this global growth hides wide inter-country variations in social media usage. In Central Asia only 6% of the population engage with social media compared to 89% in North America (We Are Social 2016). Barriers to using social media can include limitations or restrictions to access, lack of knowledge and skills or fear.

Certainly many health professionals report being fearful and wary to engage with social media (George et al. 2013).

Without the knowledge and skills needed to use social media, midwives, and other health professionals, are missing out on the advantages this method of communication and connectivity brings. Midwives and other maternity-care workers who regularly use social media have reported feeling nurtured and supported, better informed and well connected (Byrom and Byrom 2014). In addition, social media technology has broadened the scope for individuals to listen, and to voice their opinions. This has huge implications for those using and providing maternity care, as service users can share their feedback on the care they've received to the whole world, at the touch of the button. To harness the potential benefits of social media, and avoid some of the perils, health care professionals need to be provided with appropriate information, support and training so they can safely access and use social media to advance practice, respond to service-users, foster positive networks for professional development across the global stage.

In this chapter social media will be examined and explored. The benefits, challenges and possible limitations will be considered, with direct application for health professionals and health services more generally. Practical suggestions and examples will be offered to support health professionals to positively and safely engage with social media.

What Is Social Media?

Social media is the term used for a variety of internet-based digital applications that enable users to receive and share information (Kaplan and Haenlein 2010). More than 70% of UK adults who go online now have a social media profile (Ofcom 2015). Facebook, Instagram, Twitter, Snapchat and LinkedIn are amongst the popular platforms, though many others exist (see Table 9.1). Although social media channels continue to be accessed via computers and tablets, the smart phone is the device most frequently used for engaging (Ofcom 2015). It's not surprising then, that mobile apps such as Facebook Messenger and Whatsapp transmit 60 billion messages each day (Smith 2016).

Corporate industries and businesses actively and effectively use social media to market their products and services, and health care isn't excluded. Whilst there was some reticence from health care organisations in the early days of social media use, health and social care policy

Table 9.1 Social media platforms and application examples

Facebook	A popular free social networking website that allows registered users to create pro les, upload photos and video, send messages and keep in touch with friends, family and colleagues
Twitter	A social networking site that allows users to connect with each other using short messages (tweets) about any subject
Snapchat	A mobile app that allows users to capture videos and pictures that self destruct after a few seconds
LinkedIn	A business-oriented social networking service
Pinterest	A pinboard-style photo-sharing website that allows users to create and manage theme-based image collections such as events, interests, and hobbies
Instagram	An online photo-sharing, video-sharing and social networking service that enables users to take photos and videos, apply digital filters to them, and share them on a variety of social networking services
Whatsapp	A cross-platform instant-messaging application that allows smartphone users to exchange text, image, video and audio messages for free
Blogs	A discussion or informational site published on the World Wide Web and consisting of discrete entries 'posts'
Hosted chat services	Internet applications that enable live online chat, meetings and discussions.
Video sharing (YouTube, Vimeo, Animoto etc.)	A digital-imaging technology platforms that enable lms to be created/edited and shared
Research Gate	

positively encourages using digital technology to proactively engage with those whey serve (NHS England 2013). Indeed, NHS England, the Nursing and Midwifery Council, and England's Royal Colleges all use social media to share information and receive feedback. This strategy is reflected globally, with professional organisations and health departments benefiting from an online presence. On an individual level, there is still

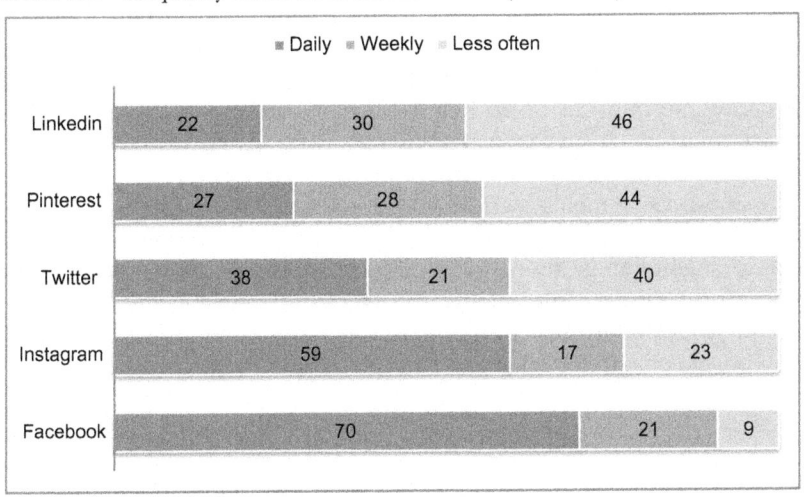

Table 9.2 Frequency of use on social media sites (Pew 2015)

Platform	Daily	Weekly	Less often
Linkedin	22	30	46
Pinterest	27	28	44
Twitter	38	21	40
Instagram	59	17	23
Facebook	70	21	9

some reluctance from health care professionals, including midwives, to take the plunge and fully embrace social media use. Fear of reprisal, lack of knowledge, and perceived lack of time all feature in the list of concerns (Byrom and Byrom 2014). Meanwhile, others report huge benefits (Ferguson 2013), and whilst it will never replace human face-to-face connection, there is huge potential for maternity services to develop social media strategies in their quest to enhance the care that women and families receive.

Navigating Social Media Platforms

As mentioned above, there are a several social media platforms to engage with (see Table 9.1). These can be accessed via desktop websites or mobile device applications. Facebook, Instagram and Twitter are the most commonly used social media networking platforms (see Table 9.2). Facebook is a virtual community and networking site, Instagram allows users to digitally enhance and share images, and Twitter is a micro-blogging application that allows users 140 characters of dialogue. All enable people to connect and interact with each other, and Facebook and Twitter provide the medium for interactive dialogues (Bagley et al. 2014). To the uninitiated, the language used by advocates of social media, may be alienating. Talk of 'platforms', 'tweeting', 'trending' and 'hashtags'—words used liberally in cyber-space—can be confusing. Specific websites such as the WeCommunities hub (2016) provide health and social care workers with a vast repository of important and useful guidance and information to help with such matters, and caters for the novice to expert. It's well worth taking a look.

Table 9.3 offers a brief glossary of terms.

As most social media platforms can link and communicate with each other in some way it has become easy, as well as important, to engage with a range of applications to create and develop an online personal or professional profile. Engaging with a range of social media platforms extends your opportunities for connection, support and impact. So what can social media do for midwives and the families they care for?

MIDWIVES AND MOTHERS—WHAT'S IN IT FOR US?

'Social media is where the future is, and most importantly, that's where our patients are going to be' (Prasad 2013).

For maternity services, we could slightly alter the above quote to *'Social media is where the future is, and most importantly, that's where the women we care for are!'* We know this to be true from various surveys, including the one by Pew (2015), which reveals that in America the most common Facebook users are women aged between 18 and 29 years (82%) and 30 and 49 years (79%). Childbearing women, and midwives, fit into these categories. The continual expansion of social media technology has maximised opportunity for individuals to be visible, accessible, and connected. This includes maternity care workers enabling them to gain and share knowledge, to build supportive networks, and to innovate.

ACCESSING SUPPORT AND SHARING KNOWLEDGE

By using social media maternity workers can access influential leaders and experts at the touch of a button, as there are no hierarchies in cyberspace (Byrom and Byrom 2014). Support for student midwives and midwives is there too, with sites such as Midwife Diaries (Durant 2016), StudentMidwife.Net (2016) and Midwives supporting Midwives (2016). Childbearing women are also using social media for information and support, and often use technology such as smartphone apps to guide

Table 9.3 Glossary of social media terms

Platforms—the various social media technologies available for us to use and engage with; examples include Facebook, Instagram, YouTube, LinkedIn
Tweet/tweeting—the micro-blog of 140 characters you can write/use on the social media platform Twitter
Handle—someone's @username on Twitter. For example, our user names are @acbmidwife and @sagefemmeSB
Hashtags (#)—these are used to tag your posts throughout social media; you can use them to target specific audiences, topics but also to help you search for specific information in most of the social media platforms, specifically, Twitter and Instagram
Apps—short for application, refers to the mobile version of social media platforms that can be downloaded on to your mobile devices, e.g., smart phoness and tablets
Avatar—An avatar is an image or username that represents a person online, most often within forums and social networks
Bio—a short piece of informative text that explains who the user is
Blog—Blog is a word that was created from two words: "web log." Blogs are usually maintained by an individual or a business with regular entries of content on a specific topic, descriptions of events, or other resources such as graphics or video
Direct Message—Direct messages (also referred to as "DMs") are private conversations that occur on Twitter. Both parties must be following one another to send a message
Forums—Also known as a message board, a forum is an online discussion site. It originated as the modern equivalent of a traditional bulletin board, and a technological evolution of the dial-up bulletin board system
Follower—In a social media setting, a follower refers to a person who subscribes to your account in order to receive your updates
Retweet—A retweet is when someone on Twitter sees your message and decides to re-share it with his or her followers. A retweet button allows them to quickly resend the message with attribution to the original sharer's name
Mention—A mention is a Twitter term used to describe an instance in which a user includes someone else's @username in their tweet to attribute a piece of content or start a discussion
Like—A Like is an action that can be made by a Facebook or Instagram user. Instead of writing a comment or sharing a post, a user can click the Like button as a quick way to show approval
Reply—A reply is a Twitter action that allows a user to respond to a tweet through a separate tweet that begins with the other user's @username. This differs from a mention, because tweets that start with an @username only appear in the timelines of users who follow both parties
Viral—used to describe an instance in which a piece of content—YouTube video, blog article, photo, etc.—achieves noteworthy awareness. Viral distribution relies heavily on word of mouth and the frequent sharing of one particular piece of content all over the internet
Vlogging—Vlogging or a vlog is a piece of content that employs video to tell a story or report on information. Vlogs are common on video-sharing networks like YouTube

them through their pregnancy, childbirth and parenting. Social media connects mothers and maternity-care workers, with an ever-increasing ability to seek and receive feedback about care. Drones are being utilized in resource poor countries, to enable much needed connectivity and information transfer via the internet (Internet.Org 2016), increasing the global reach. In Ethiopia a smartphone app has been developed to provide information to help midwives deal with emergencies. The *Safe Delivery App*, developed in Denmark, is to be distributed to 10,000 health workers across Africa and Southeast Asia by 2017 (RCM 2016). Apps are being developed and used to provide childbearing women with information too, the Baby Buddy App (Best Beginnings 2016) is free to all mothers in England, and Ask the Midwife (Harvey 2016) is a subscription-based app, available in the United Kingdom.

How to Engage—Some Guidance for Social Media Practice

Founder of WeCommunites, Teresa Chinn (2016b) believes that instead of talking about midwives and nurses using social media, the conversation should be about how to use it well. Using social media is easy, and takes just moments to set up and get going. We recommend that you find a social media role model, someone you work with that uses social media to supplement or enhance their role as a health professional. Ask if they'll show you the social media ropes, help get you started and perhaps mentor you as you navigate the range of platforms available.

Many midwives are using Facebook personally—but it's important to revisit guidance for safe and appropriate use from time to time (discussed later in this chapter). We recommend that in addition to Facebook, midwives also join Twitter. When taking the plunge to engage with the global community of midwives and midwifery matters on Twitter, you consider the following:

- When you set up your free account take care to choose a handle that reflects you; for example, you may want to use the word midwife if you are planning to join Twitter for professional benefits.
- Write an engaging bio section—read what others have written, then develop your own unique identity. This will aid others when deciding whether to follow you or not.

- Following and being followed is not the same as accepting friends on Facebook. It's more about connecting with those who share the same interests.
- When your account is set up, take a look what others are doing before tweeting if you feel unsure. You can search for key information by using the search function. Try typing in the words 'midwives', 'midwifery', 'birth', maternity' or anything you might be specifically interested in. This will help you to find people/groups to follow and read the most up-to-date tweets. When you feel more confident, join in by replying to tweets or writing your own.
- Join Tweetchats—these are organised chats, taking place on a particular date and time, usually relating to a particular topic/area of practice. They will often use a specific hashtag to help users to follow the conversation.

The WeCommunities (2016) website offers a 'Twitterversity[1]' for health care professionals from novice to expert; it's well worth a read. The site also offers a page of guidance for safe social media use, with links to resources and informative blogs.

Allaying Fears—Staying Safe with Social Media

Online blogging and digital sharing is competing with written academic articles for disseminating research and opinion, and making them more accessible. But there needs to be caution, and some health care workers lack insight of the importance of professional integrity when engaging with social media. There have been cases of inappropriate behaviour and posting on social media by some health professionals. This has led to some governing bodies producing guidance to support safe and professional use of social media.

The Nursing and Midwifery Council in the United Kingdom has developed such guidelines for nurses and midwives. Within it's guidance it stresses that 'conduct online and conduct in the real world should be judged in the same way, and should be at a similarly high standard' (NMC 2013). Chin et al. (2014) argue that the best piece of advice, with regard to professional online conduct, from the NMC is, 'If there is any

---

[1] http://www.wecommunities.org/resources/twitterversity.

doubt about whether a particular activity online is acceptable, it can be useful to think through a real-world analogy'. They suggest that before we post anything on social media, we ask ourselves whether we would post it on the staff notice board or in a room full of patients or colleagues (Chin et al. 2014). If the answer is no, then it is better not to post.

To stay safe with social media we suggest the following:

- Be clear about the privacy settings on each platform you use. Remember what you write and post can be shared with the world at the touch of a button.
- Consider whether to combine or separate personal and professional social media accounts on the various platforms.
- Respect and maintain confidentiality.
- Maintain professional boundaries at all times. Be aware of your accountability to yourself, your employer, and your professional body. Know the Code (NMC 2012).
- It's OK to observe and not participate; it's your decision.
- Model positive behaviours. Politeness is as important online as off.
- Don't engage with emotionally charged discussion. If you feel angry with a comment, move away from the situation, then consider responding. It's OK not to respond.
- Never use social media if under the influence of alcohol and other mind-altering substances.

Knowledge Translation and Mobilization

As demonstrated, social media provides health care providers, professionals, researchers and educators with extensive reach and connectivity with service-users and target audiences. Having the capacity to communicate with those in our care is an essential aspect of health care provision, research and education. Social media can be used to facilitate this communication. It is therefore a powerful tool for knowledge translation and mobilization.

It has been estimated that 80% of research evidence, relevant to clinical practice, never reaches clinicians delivering care (Glasziou 2005). A significant barrier to the translation of evidence, from demonstrated benefit into practice, is the limited time available for clinicians to search for, and appraise, emerging evidence (Lenfant 2003). Understanding both the importance of effective knowledge translation and the impact of social

Table 9.4 Benefits of social media for knowledge translation

- Speedy dissemination and exchange of information
- Broader reach
- Efficient feedback from stakeholders and target audience
- Builds communities of interest
- Easy analysis of knowledge dissemination using metric analytics
- Links target audience to primary resources
- Flexibility on when and how to deliver information/knowledge
- Enables portable content to be shared
- Encourages service-user and audience participation/collaboration
- Offers enhanced social support through social media networks

Oakley and Spallek (2012), Alberta Health Services (2016)

media in mobilizing this knowledge could have a positive impact in getting knowledge from the 'bench to the bedside' (Maloney et al. 2015).

In relation to health care, knowledge translation is defined as a dynamic and iterative process that includes the synthesis, dissemination, exchange and ethically sound application of knowledge to improve health outcomes, provide more effective health services and products and strengthen the health care system more generally. The process of translating knowledge takes place within a complex system of interactions between researchers, educators, practitioners and knowledge users which may vary in intensity, complexity and level of engagement depending on the nature of the research, education or practice as well as the needs of the particular knowledge user (Canadian Institute of Health Research 2009).

Via social media, health messages, research outcomes, training packages and practice recommendations can be disseminated rapidly and efficiently directly to specified target audiences and beyond. Table 9.4 offers an overview of the benefits of social media for knowledge translation.

However, it is important that social media channels be used to enhance traditional face-to-face knowledge dissemination rather to replace them. Combining face-to-face dissemination with social media can maximize knowledge translation, improving the impact of research, education and practice. The following sections of this chapter outline some practical ways knowledge can be shared, disseminated and translated to enhance practice and influence positive health and wellbeing outcomes. Table 9.5 Identifies key social media platforms that can help to maximize this knowledge translation.

Table 9.5 Key social media platforms for knowledge translation (KT)

Social media platform	Description	Use for KT
Twitter	A micro-blogging platform that enables users to send and read 140 character messages called tweets. These tweets can include videos, pictures and links	Increase citations (up to 20 times more citations of your peer reviewed articles—for this you do need a good following—so be a consistent and valuable user)
FaceBook	A social networking site enabling easy connections and sharing of updates, news, videos and images	Increase citations and share updates; especially using their news features, like pages and by sharing research/conference presentations using FB live (a live video-streaming function)
YouTube	It is a free video sharing website. You can watch other's videos or create and upload your own	Researchers, educators and practitioners can use YouTube to create videos (known as Vlogs —video blogs) of key messages, lessons or practice recommendations
ResearchGate	ResearchGate is a social networking site for scientists and researchers to share papers, ask and answer questions, and find collaborators. ResearchGate has over 5 million members in 193 countries. It was designed by and specifically for scientists, to meet their diverse needs, and is touted as Facebook for academics. Membership is free but is restricted to working scientists and academics (you need an academic institution email address). The major disciplines represented in ResearchGate are biology, medicine, computer science, physics, and chemistry	Researchers like using ResearchGate to be found, find others and share their work. This is one place that your work will definitely be found by potential collaborators and researchers that would like to cite your work
LinkedIn	This is a business oriented social networking service. Although it has been traditionally business oriented it contains a large number of research organisations and groups	Powerful tool for building collaborations

(continued)

Table 9.5 (continued)

Social media platform	Description	Use for KT
Academia.edu	Free sharing platform for researchers to disseminate and share their research papers	Enhances the reach, impact and citations of research

SHARED LEARNING: ONLINE CHATS AND CONFERENCES

Online chats and broadcasting from study days and conferences have added a new dimension to sharing knowledge and learning. WeCommunites (2016), comprising 16 'communities', oversees the hosting of several chats per month. @WeMidwives is part of the team, and the midwife facilitators coordinate each event, inviting interested parties to contribute to subject ideas. Whenever relevant, parents groups are invited to join in, and anyone interested in the chat are always welcomed into the conversation. A record of the chat, and those who engaged, is logged permanently on the WeCommunities website,[2] enabling participants to use the activity as evidence of ongoing professional development by using #MyWe.[3] As well as learning from others, participants are encouraged to consider the perspective of others, it maximizes potential for interacting with others globally, and the activity is free, can be undertaken at home.

Attendance at study days and events has always been a challenge for midwives, with financial and time constraints being the biggest barriers. With the advent of social media, particularly Twitter, student midwives and midwives can 'peep in' study days and conferences by following the hashtag created for the event. Non-attenders can even participate by asking questions to someone who is tweeting, which may lead to a response from a speaker. The 550 delegates who attended the Normal Labour and Birth Conference held in Sydney (Western Sydney University 2016), used the hashtag #NormalBirth16 to help share the knowledge. Using Symplur (2016) analysis the organisers were able to assess the reach, that is, the potential impact, of the event. Over the course of 3 days, the 7627 tweets had 14,339,581 impressions, and 664 individuals participated in tweeting the hashtag (so 114 more than present at the event). This is very important, as it adds value to the event.

---

[2] http://wecommunities.org.
[3] http://wecommunities.org/blogs/2177.

Persistent Activism—Creating 'Virtuous Cycles'

During a debate on the matter, Hundley and colleagues (2014) explored the potential influences of the media on the fear of childbirth. Although there is little documented evidence of a direct correlation between reality programmes such as *One Born Every Minute* and women's fear of childbirth (Hundley et al. 2015), there is frequent reporting of women informing midwives of increased anxiety after watching the programme (Butcher 2016; Garrod 2012). As with the television and press, social media provides a channel for receiving mainstream news about childbirth. This gives midwives an opportunity to try and counteract fear caused by negative reporting, by using social media to promote positive reports of childbirth. Responding to negative mainstream media is 'every midwife's business' (Byrom 2016); we must use the opportunity to challenge misinformation otherwise it allows others to define situations, and not always in the best light (McCrea 2014). A recent example of this is a blog-post response written to the publication and reporting of research relating to midwifery led care in New Zealand (Dahlen and Tracy 2016). The Positive Birth Movement, created by mother and childbirth activist Milli Hill, was created to counteract the increasing negative debates out childbirth, and to 'help change birth for the better' (PBM 2016). Via social media, Hill's global network of free-to-attend antenatal groups has expanded exponentially, and currently includes 250 groups in the United Kingdom, and over 150 in the rest of the world, including 36 different countries. This could not have been achieved without social media.

Other successful initiatives use digital platforms and co-design to engage, empower and inform those involved or interested in maternity services. #MatExp is a social movement, led by parents, families and maternity workers, and involving an innovative programme WhoseShoes© (Phillips 2016). Through various social media platforms and using the #MatExp hashtag, families, maternity care workers and activists, lawyers, academics and anyone at all interested can join together to hear, inform and lobby for change in maternity services. Instead of going round in vicious circles and continually complaining about the pressures and misgivings within maternity services, these initiatives build social media communities that enhance and interact with face-to-face workshops. By realising the mutual benefits of collaboration, relationship building and shared goals, virtuous cycles are created that facilitate positive change (Byrom and Byrom 2014).

'MIDWIFING THE MIDWIVES' THROUGH KINDNESS AND COMPASSION

With the ongoing global push for more regulated, competent and culturally aware midwives to reduce maternal and infant mortality, the need for support and encouragement is ever-present. Brodie (2013) uses the notion of 'Midwifing the Midwives' to address this, suggesting that motivation and support are crucial to recruiting and retaining midwives. Digital technology offers a global platform for this to happen; it encourages innovation and engagement, providing opportunity for radical change through building supportive networks (Byrom and Byrom 2014). The ICM's Facebook page offers a space for midwives all around the world to connect and learn. Other platforms enable individuals from different backgrounds to debate and lobby for change, if necessary. This presents exciting opportunities for collaboration and strength through maximising relationships, increasing knowledge, building virtuous cycles (Byrom and Byrom 2014) and promoting compassionate and authentic relationships (Chinn 2014). Feeling nurtured and supported is a fundamental requirement for midwives to care for others (Hunter and Warren 2015), and social media platforms such as Facebook groups or Twitter communities can help if midwives engage with like-minded others, and find their 'tribe'. Deirdre Munro's online initiative #GlobalVillageMidwives is based on promoting kindness and reciprocity, as well as offering an opportunity for learning, nurturing, encouragement and the development of friendships.

Although Chinn (2014) explores the notion that increased use of mobile technology could deter nurses and midwives from pursuing face-to-face connections, she describes how social media platforms make it easy to share our thoughts and feelings, and to respond to those of others. Chinn reminds readers of the late Dr. Kate Granger's plight to improve communication between health care workers and patients, by tweeting from her sick bed. What we witnessed on Twitter was an outpouring of love and support, and instant call to action for change using #HelloMyNameIs hashtag, which has continued since Kate's untimely death.

CONCLUSION

The ongoing maturation of social media technology has broadened the scope for individuals to be heard, and to voice their opinions. This has huge implications for those using and providing maternity care, as service users can share their feedback on the care they've received to the whole world, at the touch of the button. Online blogging is competing with written academic articles for disseminating research and opinion, and the use of social media in increasing readership of high quality papers through making them more accessible. Social media offers opportunities to maternity workers to access influential leaders and experts as there are no hierarchies in cyberspace. This in itself presents unlimited opportunities for all parties, and maximises potential for increased social capital through community engagement. It also increases visibility, the chance for student and newly qualified midwives to test out ideas, and then to gain support for taking them forwards. But there needs to be caution, and some health care professionals lack knowledge of the importance of professional integrity, and the power or demise of their digital footprint.

Editor's Note: This chapter by Byrom and Bryom clearly outlined the positives that can be yielded when midwives engage with social media. Covering a wide range of social media, the authors show how social media can encourage innovation and engagement by providing supportive networks for both clients and midwives alike. In our concluding chapter, the editor's review where this interdisciplinary field currently sits and where research needs to focus going forward.

REFERENCES

Alberta Health Services. 2016. The use of social media for knowledge translation, alberta addiction & mental health research partnership programme. Accessed at: http://www.albertahealthservices.ca/assets/info/res/mhr/if-res-mhr-kt-social-media.pdf.

Bagley, J.E., D.D. DiGiacinto, and K. Hargreaves. 2014. Imaging professionals' views of social media and its implications. *Radiologic Technology* 85 (4): 377–389.

Best Beginnings. 2016. Baby buddy app. Accessed at: https://www.bestbeginnings.org.uk/baby-buddy.

Brodie, P. 2013. Midwifing the Midwives: Addressing the empowerment, safety of, and respect for, the world's midwives. *Midwifery* 29: 1075–1076.

Byrom, S., and A. Byrom. 2014. Social media: Connection mothers and midwives globally *MIDIRS Midwifery Digest* 24 (2): 141–149.
Byrom. 2016. Accessed at: https://mediaandmidwifery.com/tag/sheena-byrom/.
Canadian Institutes of Health Research. 2009. *Social media at work: How networking tools propel organizational performance.* San Francisco: Jossey-Bass.
Chinn, T. 2014. Compassion in the social era. *The roar behind the silence: Why kindness, compassion and respect matter in maternity care.* London: Pinter and Martin.
Chinn, T. 2016a. Everything changes *Teresa Chinn Online professional community development.* Accessed at: http://teresachinn.co.uk/everything-changes/.
Chinn, T. 2016b. On a mission. *Teresa Chinn Online professional community development.* Accessed at: http://teresachinn.co.uk/on-a-mission/.
Dahlen, H., H. Dowling, M. Tracy, V. Schmied, and S. Tracy. 2013. Maternal and perinatal outcomes amongst low risk women giving birth in water compared to six birth positions on land. A descriptive cross sectional study in a birth centre over 12 years. *Midwifery* 29 (7): 759–764.
Dahlen, H. 2015. Personal communication to Sheena Byrom.
Dahlen, H., and S. Tracy. 2016. The emperors new clothes: The politics of birth research. *Thoughts of mine and others.* Accessed at: http://www.sheenabyrom.com/blog/politics—birth—research.
Durant, E. 2016. *Midwife diaries.* Accessed at: https://midwifediaries.com.
Ferguson, C. 2013. It's time for the nursing profession to leverage social media. *Journal of Advanced Nursing* 69 (4): 745–747.
Garrod, D. 2012. Birth as entertainment: What are the wider effects? *British Journal of Midwifery* 2 (2): 81.
Glasziou, P. 2005. Evidence based medicine: Does it make a difference? Make it evidence informed practice with a little wisdom. *British Medical Journal* 330 (7482): 92.
George, D., L. Rovniak, and J. Kraschnewski. 2013. Dangers and opportunities of social media for medicine. *Clinical Obstetrics and Gynaecology* 56 (3). Accessed at: Clin Obstet Gynecol. 2013 Sep; 56(3): 10.1097/GRF.0b013e318297dc38.
Harvey, H. 2016. Ask the midwife (1.0.1) [iOS]. Retrieved from https://itunes.apple.com/gb/app/id1132226644.
Hundley, V., E. van Teijlingen, and A. Luce. 2014. Fear in childbirth: Are the media responsible? *MIDIRS Midwifery Digest* 24 (4): 444–447.
Hundley, V., E. van Teijlingen, and A. Luce. 2015. Do midwives need to be more media savy? *MIDIRS Midwifery Digest* 25 (1): 5–10.
Hunter, B., and L. Warren. 2015. Caring for ourselves: The key to resilience. In *The roar behind the silence. Why kindness, compassion and respect matter in maternity care*, ed. S. Byrom and S. Downe. London: Pinter and Martin.

Internet.org. 2016. *Connecting the world.* Accessed at: https://info.internet.org/en/.

Kaplan, A.M., and M. Haenlein. 2010. Users of the world, unite! The challenges and opportunities of social media. *Business Horizons* 53: 59–68. Accessed at: http://tinyurl.com/o23ujkm.

Lenfant, C. 2003. Shattuck lecture—Clinical research to clinical practice—Lost in translation? *New England Journal of Medicine* 28, 349 (9): 868–874.

Maloney, S., J. Tunnecliff, P. Morgan, J. Giada, L. Clearihan, S. Sadasivan, et al. 2015. Translating evidence into practice via social media: A mixed-methods study. *Journal of Medical Internet Research* 17 (10). Accessed at: https://www.jmir.org/2015/10/e242.

McCrea, J.B. 2014. *On the brink of SoMething special? The first comprehensive analysis of social media in the NHS.* December 2014. Accessed at: http://jbmccrea.com/wordpress/wp-content/uploads/2014/12/State-of-Social-Media-in-the-NHS.pdf.

Midwives Supporting Midwives. 2016. Accessed at: https://www.facebook.com/groups/733404866734223/.

NHS England. 2103. Transforming participation in health and care. Accessed at: https://www.england.nhs.uk/wp-content/uploads/2013/09/trans-part-hc-guid1.pdf.

Nursing and Midwifery Council. 2013. *Applying the code to the use of social networking sites.* http://www.nmc-uk.org/Nurses-and-midwives/Advice-by-topic/A/Advice/Social-networking-sites/.

Oakley, M., and H. Spallek. 2012. Social media in dental education: A call for research and action. *Journal of Dental Education* 76 (3): 279–287.

Ofcom. 2015. *Adults media use and attitudes report* http://stakeholders.ofcom.org.uk/market-data-research/other/research-publications/adults/media-lit-10years/.

Patient Opinion. 2016. *Patient opinion.* Accessed at: https://www.patientopinion.org.uk.

Phillips G. 2016. Whose shoes? Accessed at: http://nutshellcomms.co.uk.

Prasad, B. 2013. Social media, health care and social networking. *Gastrointestinal Endoscopy* 77 (3): 492–495.

Positive Birth Movement. 2016. *Welcome to the positive birth movement.* Accessed at: http://www.positivebirthmovement.org.

Royal College of Midwives. 2016. App for emergencies. *Midwives* 19: 14.

Smith, K. 2016. Marketing: 96 amazing social media statistics and facts for 2016 *brandwatch.* Accessed at: https://www.brandwatch.com/2016/03/96-amazing-social-media-statistics-and-facts-for-2016/.

StudentMidwife.Net. 2016. Accessed at: https://studentmidwife.net.

Symplur. 2016. *Strengthening the quiet voices in healthcare.* Accessed at: http://www.symplur.com.
We Are Social. 2016. We are social. Accessed at: http://wearesocial.com.
WeCommunites. 2016. *WeMidwives.* http://www.wenurses.com/about/index.php.
Wernham, E., J. Gurney, J. Stanley, L. Ellison-Loschmann, and D. Sarfati. 2016. A comparison of midwife-led and medical-led models of care and Their relationship to adverse fetal and neonatal outcomes: A retrospective cohort study in New Zealand. *PLoS Med* 13 (9): e1002134.
Western Sydney University. 2016. 11th international normal labour and birth conference. Accessed at: https://www.westernsydney.edu.au/nursingandmidwifery/home/news-and-events/2016NLBC.

CONCLUSIONS

Keywords Midwifery · Media · Discourse · Health professionals Practitioners

The journey to produce this book started with a chance discussion between a midwifery researcher, Prof. Vanora Hundley, and an academic journalist, Dr. Ann Luce. Frustrated with the limited impact that midwifery interventions were having to reduce early hospital admission in the latent phase of labour, Hundley brought together the team that includes renowned sociologist Prof. Edwin van Teijlingen to look at whether a societal intervention might be the answer. Rather than creating the much hoped for intervention, the result was a slightly heated discussion about whose responsibility it was for the unrealistic portrayals of childbirth.

This discussion subsequently translated into a public engagement event with support from the National Childbirth Trust's, Elizabeth Duff and frequent BBC Radio pundit Joanne Dewberry, co-founder of Networking Mummies (Hundley et al. 2014). This event, attended by more than 50 midwives and midwifery academics, led to our systematic review (Luce et al. 2016). We wanted to see what was already published in the field, and we did not find much! After an initial keyword search yielded more than 4000 publications, we whittled that systematically down to just 38, with 20 pieces of published or non-published quantitative, qualitative or mixed-method approaches, while the remaining 18 were grey literature. We determined that childbirth is depicted as being medicalised, risky, dangerous—something to be feared; that the media is the dominant way for women to learn about childbirth; and, lastly, that in the media birth is missing as a 'normal' everyday life event (Luce et al. 2016).

We began to build a body of work: the systematic review led us to wonder if midwives knew how to engage with media, so we hosted a workshop and taught midwives how to talk to journalists. Discussions that emerged in that workshop led to the consideration of creating media guidelines for both midwives and media producers, something Luce (WHO 2008, 2017; SAVE 2017) has had much experience with in working in the field of suicide prevention. What also emerged from that workshop was the fear that traditional media and social media evoked in midwives (Hundley et al. 2015). In response, we conducted some research, the findings of which you have already read in Chap. 7 of this book (Luce et al. 2017). We also wondered how social media was used by both pregnant women and midwives; these findings are forthcoming in a journal article. But all the while, we kept coming back to the question of how to change the narrative around childbirth and whose responsibility is it. That question led us to put together this book.

We wanted to bring some of the finest scholars who have been researching in the area of media and midwifery together to share their thoughts about what they have found and where they feel our collective research agenda should focus. We wanted to move the conversation forward. We believe we have done this; yet more work needs to be done.

The research team of Hundley, van Teijlingen and Luce will continue to work on the challenges of supporting women in the latent phase of labour, but we are currently fascinated by changing the discourse around childbirth and early labour—we are not even sure if it can be done, but we are going to try.

We have secured a Ph.D. studentship at Bournemouth University to try and tackle this subject from multiple perspectives (the woman's, midwives' and the media's). In this research, the Ph.D. candidate is going to conduct a discourse analysis of newspapers and television to determine the common discourses around childbirth and early labour. Focus groups with women and families will help us determine how media representations of labour and birth are interpreted, while interviews with media producers will establish whether it is possible to harness the media to correct misinformation and change discourses around labour and birth. The aim is to create a media intervention that can be used, in the same way as Luce's work on suicide, to improve how childbearing is approached by the media.

CONCLUSIONS 151

What we have determined and now accept, based on our body of work, is that the two professions of media and midwifery may seem to be unlikely bedfellows; indeed, they are often reported to be at loggerheads with one another, yet the two MUST work together to get this narrative right. We have seen from our contributing authors, Maclean (Chap. 3), Angell (Chap. 4), and Dahlen (Chap. 8) that horror stories that often make for graphic reading tend to have significant long-term effects on the health of mothers and babies. They distance women from normal birth, as explored by Maclean in Chap. 3; create fear, as discussed by Leachman in Chap. 5, and put women off feeding their babies in the way that is best for their health, according to Angell in Chap. 4. It could be argued that the media has a responsibility for ethical and responsible reporting; after all, such guidelines exist with regard to suicide (WHO 2008, 2017; SAVE 2017). However, what we are discussing here is *journalistic representation of midwifery*. Accessing correct information requires professional input and it is here that midwives have a moral responsibility, as discussed by Luce et al. in Chap. 7; Dahlen in Chap. 8 and Byrom and Byrom in Chap. 9.

The role the media plays, or should play, in the dissemination of information to women remains a challenge for health professionals. Women, according to Roberts et al. in Chap. 2, are turning to television for information on childbirth while access to antenatal education is declining. Midwives may feel this is an inappropriate role for the media, as we have seen in the chapter by Luce et al. (Chap. 7). However, Rodger et al. argue, in Chap. 6, that more can be done by midwives to engage pregnant women online and through the use of health applications on their mobile phones. Guidelines for responsible representations of midwifery in television programming may need to be explored, as well as best practice for engaging women in a clinical environment.

Over the last several years, we have thoroughly debated these topics in classrooms, at symposia, workshops, through stakeholder events and engagement with the general public. We believe that no one profession can move forward the agenda to change the discourse around childbirth. Midwives and media producers MUST work together, must learn from each other and must respect each other in order for change to happen.

It is important for midwives to engage with media producers and journalists to help improve the representation of childbirth both in journalism and on television. This can be seen, for example, in the popular BBC programme *Call the Midwife*. This is significantly different from other fictional portrayals of childbirth on TV because of the midwifery adviser input from the outset (see Roberts et al. in Chap. 2). It is also just as important for media producers and journalists to listen to midwives to understand the negative implications dramatic and risky narratives can have on pregnant women and their babies. The challenge we face now is how best to get these two fields to work together to engage both midwives and media producers in this respect.

Both of these fields yield practitioners, a common starting point. Media practitioners are storytellers and are good communicators, while midwives excel at providing care and support. A re-contextualisation of these fields is needed. This will require a commitment to open-mindedness, flexibility and co-operation. We need to conceptualise old problems in new and innovative ways.

Together, these two ostensibly incommensurate disciplines should dialogue and combine in new, exciting and valuable ways in order to forge a *new* field of practice; and, of course, of theory, philosophy and new ways of thinking of media and midwifery.

Index

A
Abortion, 28
Abrahams, S.W., 47
Academia.edu, 141
Adams, S.S., 28
Adorno, T., 17
Age, The (newspaper), 26
Agutter, J., 35, 37
Ajayi, I.O., 82, 88
Allan, S., 24, 26, 29
Amu, O., 80
Andrew, N., 47
Angell, C., 4, 50, 54, 151
Antenatal clinic, 80, 81, 83, 85–88, 90
Apps (software applications), 82, 91, 92, 131, 133, 135
Asbeek Brusse, E.D., 15
Ashe, D., 81
Ask the Midwife (app), 136
Aslama, M., 15
Association for Improvements in the Maternity Services, 15
Australian College of Midwives, 4
Autopsies, 15

B
Baby buddy app, 136
Bagley, J.E., 133
Bamgboye, E.A., 82, 88
Banet-Weiser, S., 16
Bariatric surgery, 41, 42
Barker, K., 10, 13
Bartick, M., 46
Baumeister, R., 117
Beautiful Births Documentary, 69
Beck, U., 27, 30, 31
Behind the Headlines (NHS webpage), 24
Benefit Street, 16
Bergmann, R.L., 52
Betts, D., 122, 123
Bick, D., 27, 115
Biressi, A., 17
'Birthporn', 16
Blogs, 9, 74, 112, 118, 120, 122, 125, 135, 137, 140, 142
Boden, G., 13, 15
'Born before arrival' (BBA) births, 32
Boulton, T., 18

© The Editor(s) (if applicable) and The Author(s) 2017
A. Luce et al. (eds.), *Midwifery, Childbirth and the Media*,
DOI 10.1007/978-3-319-63513-2

Bournemouth University, 2, 4
Boyer, K., 54
Bramwell, R., 47
Breastfeeding
   and academic research, 47
   depicted as comedy, 52
   depicted as normal behaviour, 52
   depiction of health risks and benefits, 53
   difficulties with, 52
   and media messaging, 50, 51
   and media stereotyping, 51
   and positive birth experience, 73
   and public gaze, 54
   and public opinion, 47
   recommendations for, 46
   and social trends, 49
   statistics, 87
Brett, M., 16, 17
Bridges, N., 48, 50, 55
Brocklehurst, P., 28, 34
Brodie, P., 143
Brook, J., 80
Brossard, D., 48
Brown, J.D., 48, 52–54
Buse, K., 28
Business of Being Born, The (documentary), 69
Bylaska-Davies, P., 50, 55
Byrom, A., 5, 131, 133, 134, 143
Byrom, S., 5, 131, 133, 134, 143

C
Caesarean section
   and cascade of intervention, 27
   cost of, 73
   elective, 26, 28, 62, 71
   emergency, 10, 28, 32, 35
   and fear of childbirth, 10, 11
   and media depictions of labour and birth, 116
   morbidity, 116
   repeat, 122
   rising rate of, 25, 98
   vaginal birth after, 122
Call the Midwife (television series), 37, 118, 151
Caplice, S., 98
Carter, S.K., 48
'Cascade of intervention', 27, 31
Casualty (television series), 13
Chamberlain, Z., 16
Cheng, Y.W., 30
Chezem, J., 47
Childbirth, 2. *See also* Caesarean section; Fear of childbirth; Labour; Pregnancy
   'born before arrival' (BBA) births, 33
   and 'delivery', 26, 34, 136
   home birth, 33, 34, 38, 62, 65, 73
   hospital birth, 73
   and maternal position, 16
   medicalisation of, 26, 101, 115
   myths of, 65, 70
   'perfect representation' of, 4, 19
   as 'women's business', 99, 118
Chinn, T., 136, 143
Clement, S., 99
Clifft-Matthews, V., 12
Cockington, R.A., 81
Conboy, M., 24
Conversation, The (media outlet), 118, 126
Coxon, K., 26, 27, 30
Cumberledge, J., 24, 29

D
Dahlen, H., 4, 26, 69, 76, 98, 113, 116, 117, 120, 121, 127, 142
Daily Express (newspaper), 35, 36
Daily Mail (newspaper), 26, 33, 38

Daily Mirror (newspaper), 37
Daily Telegraph (newspaper), 25, 32, 36, 115
Das, S., 80
De Benedictis, S., 3, 14, 16
Declercq, E.R., 98
De la Vega, R., 92
Desmarais, S.L., 27
Dewberry, J., 149
Dhulkotia, J.S., 80
Dick-Read, G., 28, 32
Discourse, 2, 9
  gendered discourse, 18
  and infant feeding, 47, 53
  of medicine, 121
  as social practice, 9
  and television, 15, 16
Dodgson, J.E., 48–50, 52, 53
Domestic violence, 99
Donnison, J., 28, 99
Dore, M., 13
Dovey, J., 14
Duff, E., 149
Durant, E., 134
Duvall, S.-S., 48, 51, 55
Dworkin, S., 26

E
Ehrenreich, B., 29
English, E., 29
Epidurals, 35, 36, 76, 115
Eriksson, C., 101
Evening Standard (newspaper), 25, 29

F
Facebook, 13, 70, 75, 105, 107, 108, 119, 131, 133, 135, 136, 140, 143. *See also* Social media
Farrell, N., 29, 34, 35
Fear *See* Fear of childbirth

Fear of childbirth
  and adverse outcomes, 28
  and caesarean section, 2, 10, 28
  fear of losing control, 72
  fear of losing dignity and respect, 72
  fear of pain, 71
  media's use of psychology of fear, 117
  occurrence of, 10
  and *One Born Every Minute*, 8
  and planning for birth, 10
  and prolonged labour, 28
  tokophobia, 10, 29, 32, 62
Fear Free Childbirth (podcast), 4, 63
Fenwick, J., 10, 28
Fetal heart monitor, 27
Film *See* Television and film
Formula milk feeding, 49–53. *See also* Infant feeding
Foss, K.A., 48, 49, 51–53
Foucault, M., 27
Framing, 25, 29, 48, 123, 125
Frazier, L., 47
Frerichs, L., 52
Furness, H., 13

G
Galtung, J., 24, 33
Gardham, D., 115
Gardner, D., 116
Garrod, D., 10, 12, 14, 18, 142
Gastric bypass surgery, 32
Gauntlett, D., 11
George, D., 131
Gibbons, K, 81
Gibson, R., 26
Gignon, M., 82
Gilchrist, L., 36
Gill, R., 9, 14
Glasziou, P., 138

#GlobalVillageMidwives (online initiative), 143
Granger, K., 143
Grauer, A., 10
Greer, J., 10
Guardian, The (newspaper), 25, 27, 32, 34
Gutteridge, K., 101

H
Haenlein, M., 131
Haines, H., 28
Hall, A., 12
Hamad, H., 8, 14
Hamilton, A.E., 48, 55
Harcup, T., 24
Harvey, H., 136
Harvey, K., 47
Hashtags, 134, 135. *See also* Social media
Hauck, Y., 80
Hausman, B.L., 53
Hayter, M., 107
Headlines, 4, 24–26, 28–33, 35, 36, 65, 67, 69, 114, 115, 124
Health-e Baby project, 80
Health promotion strategies, 80–82, 85
  and competing interests, 89
  and information needs and preferences, 89, 92
  mobile phones, 90
  posters and pamphlets, 85
  and waiting room waiting time, 87, 89
Heaton, M., 35
#HelloMyNameIs (online initiative), 143
Henderson, A., 48, 49, 51, 53
Hill, M., 8, 142
Hoddinott, P., 46

Hofberg, K., 28
Holmes, S., 16, 17
Home birth, 33, 34, 38, 62, 65, 73
Homer, C., 26, 120, 121
Hooper, C., 37
Horn, M.S., 81, 82
Horta, B.L., 46
Houghton, G., 27
Houston, W., 113, 114
Howes, V., 13
Hundley, V., 98, 99, 102, 142
Hunter, B., 143

I
Independent (newspaper), 25
Infant feeding, 4. *See also* Breastfeeding
  formula milk feeding, 46, 49–56
  and health risks and benefits, 53, 54
  media coverage of, 47–55
  and media messaging, 50, 51
  and media stereotyping, 51
  and social trends,, 49, 50
Ingram, J., 47
Instagram, 112, 118, 131, 133, 135. *See also* Social media
International Day of the Midwife, 121
Internet discussion forums, 112, 122

J
Jackson, C.J., 80
Janssen, P.A., 27
Jarallah, J.S., 82, 88
Jensen, T., 16
Jermyn, D., 16, 17
John, B., 106
Johnson, R., 28
Jones, C., 107
Jordan, B., 121
Journal of Clinical Nursing, 107

K
Kakuma, R., 46
Kaplan, A.M., 131
Kelly, Y., 51
Kennedy, H.P., 115
Khan, R., 32
Kildea, S., 81
Kingdon, C., 25, 26
Kitzinger, S., 36
Klass, M., 36
Kline, K.N., 12
Knight, M., 31
Kramer, M.S., 46
Kraschnewski, J.L., 92

L
Labour
 early labour, 2, 3
 and epidurals, 35, 36, 74, 76, 115
 fast labour, 32
 and fear, 10, 28, 69, 71, 103
 and headlines, 24, 31, 32
 and lack of support,, 11
 and midwifery, 12–14, 108
 normalising of, 32
 and pain, 15, 16, 25, 33, 35, 36, 62, 63, 71, 101, 115
 prolonged labour, 10, 28
 and risk perception, 27
 and women's magazines, 26
Lacey, N., 27
Laja, S., 100
Lancaster, P., 35
Larsson, M., 28
Laursen, M.C., 10
Lavender, T., 10
Leachman, A., 4, 10, 17
Lenfant, C., 138
Leong, Z.A., 81, 82, 91
Leveson, B., 24
Lewis, M., 48, 55

Light, E.C., 46
LinkedIn, 131, 135, 140. *See also* Social media
Loewenstein, G., 27, 31
Longhurst, R., 15
Lothian, J.A., 10
Louis XIV of France, 66
Low, N.B., 81
Luce, A., 11, 26, 37, 98, 102, 115
Lupton, D., 24, 30
Lylerly, A.D., 18

M
Maclean, E., 4, 25, 37, 38, 98
Macnamara, J., 50
Madden, R., 82, 83
Mail on Sunday (newspaper), 31, 35
Malacrida, C., 18
Maloney, S., 139
Mannien, J., 47, 50, 54, 55
#MatExp (social movement), 142
McAndrew, F., 46
McCombs, M., 50
McCrea, J.B., 142
McGrath, B.M., 81
McKee, A., 18
McNiel, M.E., 53
Media, 4. *See also* Newspapers; Podcasts; Social media; Television and film
 and birth education, 69
 and health promotion strategies, 80–82, 84–91, 93
 and infant feeding, 46–51, 53, 55
 and midwives, 12–14, 24–30, 32–36, 38, 101, 120, 121
Media effects model, 11
Media engagement, 37
 and 'bad is stronger than good', 117
 and changing discourse, 100, 102
 and distrust of media, 102, 104

and drama, 114–116
and humility, 113, 114
and midwives, 98, 100–108, 112–115, 117–121, 124, 127
and patience, 113
and persistence, 113
practical tips, 124
and resilience, 111–114
social media, 4
and twitchers, 116
and universities, 118
Media releases, 118, 124
Media training, 38, 106, 107
Medicalisation of childbirth, 3, 10, 26, 28, 69, 71, 101, 115
Mental health, 28, 73, 87
Metro (newspaper), 25
Miah, A., 15
Microbirth (documentary), 69
Midwife Diaries (website), 134
Midwifery
 and academic literature, 98, 101
 and antenatal clinic, 83, 84
 and changing discourse through media, 100
 and distrust of media, 103
 and engagement with media, 4, 98
 media depictions of, 116
 and media training, 106, 107
 and newspapers, 24–27, 29, 33, 36, 37
 and reality television, 9, 10, 12, 16, 17
 and social media, 104–108, 131, 134, 136, 138, 139, 141, 144
Midwifing the Midwives, 143
Midwives Supporting Midwives (website), 134
Miro, J., 92
Miscarriage, 123
Mobile and smart phones
 apps, 82, 91, 92, 131, 133, 135

and health promotion strategies, 85, 88, 90, 91
and social media, 130, 134, 136
Mohamad, E., 48
Montazeri, A., 81
Morris, C., 47, 51
Morse, J.M., 84
Mostyn, T., 47
Munro D., 143
Munro, S., 11
Murphy-Lawless, J., 117
Murphy, R., 81
Murray, J., 35

N
Nairn, S., 13
Narain, J., 51
National Childbirth Trust, 149
National Collaborating Centre for Women's and Children's Health, 12
National Health Service (NHS), 13, 24, 28, 29, 33, 37, 99, 101, 132
National Maternity Review, 29
Neilsen, J., 31
Newspapers
 broadsheet language, 30, 36
 and celebrity births, 35, 36
 'freak' stories, 32
 headlines, 4, 25, 28, 29, 31–33, 35, 36
 and home births, 33
 and infant death, 52
 and infant feeding, 46–50, 52–55
 and midwives, 25, 26, 28, 29, 32, 36
 practical tips for dealing with, 124, 127
 and pregnancy complications, 31
 and tabloid language, 36
 and traumatic births, 35

Ngoc, T.V., 91
Nolan, M., 27
Normal Labour and Birth Conference, 141
Nunn, H., 17
Nursing and Midwifery Council, 12, 99, 105, 132, 137

O
Oakley, M., 139
O'Brien, E., 49, 50, 52–55
O'Brien Hill, G.E., 15, 16
Obstetricians, 26, 30, 32, 112, 119, 120
Odent, M., 28
One Born Every Minute (reality television show), 3, 35, 36, 68, 75, 101, 102, 115, 142
O'Neill, D., 24
Online chats and conferences, 141
O'Reilly, K., 83
Orr, L., 99
Otley, H., 101

P
Page, L., 11
Pain
 and breastfeeding, 51
 and childbirth, 15, 16, 26, 35, 64, 65, 71, 102, 115
 fear of, 71, 101
 female pain as entertainment, 15, 16
 gendered pain, 16
 and miscarriage, 123
 pain-free childbirth, 62
Pantti, M., 16
Parenting magazines and websites, 126
Parry, K., 47
Peuchaud, S.R., 48, 52–54
Phillips, G., 142

Phones. *See* Mobile and smart phones
Podcasts, 63, 74, 75
Portwood-Stacer, L., 16
Positive Birth Movement, 142
Potter, B., 48, 49, 52
'Poverty porn', 16
Prasad, B., 104, 134
Pre-eclampsia, 29, 31
Pregnancy, 4. *See also* Childbirth; Midwifery
 and bariatric surgery, 241, 242
 'convenience pregnancy', 26
 and fear of childbirth, 10
 and health promotion practices, 80–82, 84–86, 88, 89
 medical complications, 31
 miscarriage, 123
 and public domain, 118
 and social media/technology, 106, 108, 119, 134
Public health, 15, 25, 28, 46

R
Radio, 75, 76, 112, 114, 119, 125
Reah, D., 33
Reality television, 9–12, 16, 17. *See also One Born Every Minute* (reality television show)
 definition of, 17
 and genre, 17
 and impact on childbirth experience, 10
 and realism, 18
Reese, S.D., 50
Reinhold, A., 46
Renfrew, M.J., 25, 28
ResearchGate, 140
Richens, Y., 10
Rich, P.R., 28
Riddoch, L., 99
Riordan, J., 52

Risk perception, 25, 27
Risk society, 27
Roberts, J., 3, 5, 15
Robson, S., 26
Rodger, D., 4, 83, 91, 93
Rodriguez-Garcia, R., 47
Rogers, J., 13
Rossignol, M., 27
Rothman, B.K., 18
Rouhe, H., 28
Rowe, K., 53
Royal College of Midwives (RCM), 11, 14, 32, 38, 98, 99, 104, 136
Royal College of Obstetricians and Gynaecologists (RCOG), 32
Ruge, M.H., 33

S
Safe Delivery App, 136
Sajadian, A., 81
Sandall, J., 28
Scamell, M., 27, 30, 32
Schroeder, E., 73
Schwitzer, G., 99
Scott, B.J., 47
Scott, J., 47
Seale, C., 49, 116
Seddon, E., 13, 14
Shaikh, U., 47
Shennan, A.H., 31
Shoemaker, P.J., 50
Simonsen, S.E., 15
Skeggs, B., 9, 12, 17
Skuse, A., 4
Sky News, 38
Slade, P., 28
Sloan, S., 46
Smart phones. *See* Mobile and smart phones
Smith, K., 131
Social media
  and academic institutions, 14, 48
  cautions for, 100, 130, 144
  defined, 130, 131
  Facebook, 13, 70, 75, 105, 107, 108, 119, 131, 133–136, 140, 143
  fear of, 98
  guidance for social media practice, 136
  and health care organisations, 131
  and infant feeding, 47, 48
  Instagram, 112, 118, 119, 131, 133, 135
  knowledge translation and mobilization, 138–140
  and midwifery, 3–5, 4, 98–100, 103–106, 108, 109, 111, 112, 127, 130–132, 134, 136, 137, 140, 150
  platforms, 132
  and safety, 136–138
  as source of support and knowledge, 118
  statistics, 27
  terminology, 17
  Twitter, 105, 108, 112, 119, 131, 133, 135, 136, 140, 141, 143
Spiby, H., 3
Stapleton, H., 81
Stereotyping
  and childbirth, 102
  and infant feeding, 51, 53
  and media discourse, 4
Stewart, R., 35
Stillbirth, 29, 31
StudentMidwife.Net, 134
Stuthridge, T., 15
Suicide, 99
Sun (newspaper), 25, 31, 32, 34, 35
Sundar, S.S., 26
Sunday Express (newspaper), 29
Sunday Times (newspaper), 30, 31

T

Taylor, M., 103
Television and film
  and childbirth, 2, 8, 10–16, 18, 19
  and discourse analysis, 9, 14, 15, 17, 18
  as education, 16–18
  as entertainment, 14–16
  and health promotion programs, 81
  and infant feeding, 47, 48, 51–53, 55, 56
  and midwives, 12–14, 101, 120, 121
  One Born Every Minute, 3, 8–16, 18, 19, 35, 36, 68, 75, 101, 102, 115, 118, 142
  practical tips for, 124
  and 'talent', 114, 126
Tempier, R.P., 81
Templeton, S.K., 30
Thomson, G., 11, 47
Times, The (newspaper), 25, 30
Timmons, S., 13
Tokophobia (extreme fear of childbirth), 10, 29, 32, 62. *See also* Fear of childbirth
Tracy, M., 28, 31
Tracy, S., 28, 31, 142
Tuckett, A., 107
Tulloch, J., 24, 30
Turner, C., 107
24 Hours in A&E (television documentary series), 13
Twitter, 105, 108, 112, 119, 131, 133, 135, 136, 140, 141, 143. *See also* Social media
Tyler, I., 16

U

Ultrasound exams, 15
UNICEF, 46, 82

Unterscheider, J., 33

V

Van Esterik, P., 48, 53, 54
Van Teijlingen, E., 2, 3, 37, 98, 99, 142, 149, 150
Vaughan, W., 15
Victora, C.G., 46
Vlogging, 135

W

Wachs, F., 26
Waiting rooms, 80–82, 85, 88, 91, 93
Wall, G., 47
Walsh, D., 114, 115
Wambach, K., 52
Ward, K., 81
Ward, M.R., 28
Warren, L., 143
Watt, R., 51
WeCommunities (website), 134, 137, 141
Whitbread, F., 35
Wicke, D.M., 81
Wilmore, M., 4, 87
Wood, H., 12, 17
World Health Organisation (WHO), 46, 81
Wylie, L., 105

Y

Young, M., 27
YouTube, 135, 140

Z

Zelizer, B., 26
Zhang, Y., 49
Zillman, D., 26

Printed by Printforce, the Netherlands